Volume 01
Issue 03
November 2006

# The Senses & Society

BERG

## AIMS AND SCOPE

A heightened interest in the role of the senses in culture and society is sweeping the human sciences, supplanting older paradigms and challenging conventional theories of representation.

This pioneering journal provides a crucial forum for the exploration of this vital new area of inquiry. It brings together groundbreaking work in the humanities and social sciences and incorporates cutting-edge developments in art, design, and architecture. Every volume contains something for and about each of the senses, both singly and in all sorts of novel configurations.

Sensation is fundamental to our experience of the world. Shaped by culture, gender, and class, the senses mediate between mind and body, idea and object, self and environment. The senses are increasingly extended beyond the body through technology, and catered to by designers and marketers, yet persistently elude all efforts to capture and control them. Artists now experiment with the senses in bold new ways, disrupting conventional canons of aesthetics.

- How is perception shaped by cultures and technologies?
- In what ways are the senses sites for the production and practice of ideologies of gender, class, and race?
- How many senses are there to "aesthetics"?
- What are the social implications of the increasing commercialization of sensation?
- How might a focus on the cultural life of the senses yield new insights into processes of cognition and emotion?

*The Senses & Society* aims to:

- Explore the intersection between culture and the senses
- Promote research on the politics of perception and the aesthetics of everyday life
- Address architectural, marketing, and design initiatives in relation to the senses
- Publish reviews of books and multi-sensory exhibitions throughout the world
- Publish special issues concentrating on particular themes relating to the senses

To submit an article, please write to Michael Bull at:

The Senses and Society
Department of Media & Film Studies
University of Sussex
Brighton
Sussex
BN1 9QQ
UK

email:
senses@sussex.ac.uk or
m.bull@sussex.ac.uk

Books for review should be sent to David Howes at:

The Senses and Society
Department of Sociology and Anthropology
Concordia University
1455 de Maisonneuve Boulevard West
Montreal, Quebec
H3G 1M8
CANADA

email:
senses@alcor.concordia.ca
howesd@vax2.concordia.ca

Comments and suggestions regarding Sensory Design reviews should be addressed to Joy Monice Malnar

email:
malnar@uiuc.edu

Comments and suggestions regarding multisensory exhibition and conference reviews should be addressed to Bill Arning

email:
barning@mit.edu

©2006 Berg. All rights reserved.
No part of this publication may be reproduced or utilized in any form or by any means, electronic or mechanical, including photocopying and recording, or by any information storage or retrieval system, without permission in writing from the publisher.

ISSN: 1745-8927

## SUBSCRIPTION INFORMATION

Three issues per volume.

One volume per annum.

2006: Volume 1

ONLINE
www.bergpublishers.com

BY MAIL
Berg Publishers
C/o Customer Services
Turpin Distribution
Pegasus Drive
Stratton Business Park
Biggleswade
Bedfordshire SG18 8TQ
UK

BY FAX
+44 (0)1767 601640

BY TELEPHONE
+44 (0)1767 604951

BY EMAIL
custserv@turpin-distribution.com

INQUIRIES

Kathryn Earle, Managing Editor
email: kearle@bergpublishers.com

Production: Ian Critchley, email:
icritchley@bergpublishers.com

Advertising and subscriptions:
Veruschka Selbach,
email: vselbach@bergpublishers.com

SUBSCRIPTION RATES

Institutions' subscription rate
£155/US$289

Individuals' subscription rate
£40/US$70*

*This price is available only to personal subscribers and must be prepaid by personal cheque or credit card

Free online subscription for institutional subscribers

Full color images available online

Access your electronic subscription through www.ingenta.com

REPRINTS FOR MAILING

Copies of individual articles may be obtained from the publishers at the appropriate fees.
Write to
Berg Publishers
1st Floor, Angel Court
81 St Clements Street
Oxford OX4 1AW
UK

## Founding Editors

Michael Bull and David Howes

## EDITORIAL BOARD

### Managing Editor

Michael Bull, University of Sussex, UK

### Editors

Paul Gilroy, *London School of Economics, UK*

David Howes, *Concordia University, Canada*

Douglas Kahn, *University of California, Davis, USA*

### Sensory Design Editor

Joy Monice Malnar, *University of Illinois, Urbana-Champaign*

### Book Reviews Editor

David Howes, *Concordia University*

### Exhibition and Conference Reviews Editor

Bill Arning, *Massachusetts Institute of Technology, USA*

## ADVISORY BOARD

Alison Clarke, *University of Vienna, Austria*

Steven Connor, *University of London, UK*

Alain Corbin, *Université de Paris I, La Sorbonne, France*

Ruth Finnegan, *Open University, UK*

Jukka Gronow, *University of Uppsala, Sweden*

Peter Charles Hoffer, *University of Georgia, USA*

Caroline Jones, *Massachusetts Institute of Technology, USA*

Barbara Kirshenblatt-Gimblett, *New York University, USA*

Margaret Morse, *University of California at Santa Cruz, USA*

Ruth Phillips, *Carleton University, Canada*

Leigh Schmidt, *Princeton University, USA*

Mark Smith, *University of South Carolina, USA*

Jonathan Sterne, *McGill University, Canada*

Paul Stoller, *West Chester University, USA*

Michael Syrotinski, *University of Aberdeen, UK*

Nigel Thrift, *University of Oxford, UK*

Fran Tonkiss, *London School of Economics, UK*

Typeset by JS Typesetting Ltd, Porthcawl, Mid Glamorgan
Printed in the UK

**The Senses & Society**

**Volume 01
Issue 03
November 2006**

# Contents

### Articles

293  **Fantasy Lands and Kinesthetic Thrills: Sensorial Consumption, the Shock of Modernity and Spectacle as Total-Body Experience at Coney Island**
Lynn Sally

311  **The Sensory Dimensions of Gardening**
Christopher Tilley

331  **Learning How To Listen: Kroncong Music in a Javanese Neighborhood**
Steve Ferzacca

359  **The Anti-Pod**
Kathleen Ferguson

### Sensory Design

369  **Restorative Bath Waters: Bath Spa, Bath, England**
Christie Pearson

373  **The LDS Conference Center**
William C. Miller and Ryan E. Smith

### Book Reviews

381  **Cross-talk between the Senses**
  Gemma Calvert, Charles Spence and Barry E. Stein (eds.), *The Handbook of Multisensory Processes*
  *Visual Music: Synaesthesia in Art and Music Since 1900*, with contributions by Kerry Brougher, Olivia Mattis, Jeremy Strick, Ari Wiseman and Judith Zilzcer
  Reviewed by David Howes

**391**   **A Sense of Things to Come: On the Emergent Dialogue between Contemporary Art and Anthropology**
      Arnd Schneider and Christopher Wright, eds., *Contemporary Art and Anthropology*
        Reviewed by Andrew Irving

## Exhibition and Conference Reviews

**399**   **Even-handedness**
      "The Prisoners' Inventions"
        Reviewed by Kevin Henry

**405**   **Synesthesia Soirées**
      "Four Soirées around the Theme of Synaesthesia"
        Reviewed by Maaike Bleeker

**409**   **Senses of Identity**
      "A Sense of Identity"
        Reviewed by Willow Sainsbury and Danny George

# Fantasy Lands and Kinesthetic Thrills
## Sensorial Consumption, the Shock of Modernity and Spectacle as Total-Body Experience at Coney Island

### Lynn Sally

Lynn Sally received her Ph.D. from the Performance Studies Department at New York University in 2004. This article expands on a chapter in her dissertation, "Fighting the Flames: The Spectacular Performance of Fire at Coney Island," forthcoming from Routledge Press. lsally@metropolitan.edu.

ABSTRACT This article proposes that Coney Island's enclosed amusement parks aided in the transformation of spectacle as total-body experience. By studying the ways that Coney Island's unique beachside resort produced entertainment that appealed to all of the senses, we seek to "make sense" of the amusement area in its historical and geographic specificity. Even in its early years of development the beachside resort was touted (and critiqued) in the popular press as a carnivalesque atmosphere that escalated the senses. With the opening of Steeplechase, Luna Park and Dreamland Coney Island's enclosed amusement parks provided dream worlds of technological and architectural wonder that invited the consumption of leisure as participatory and kinesthetic. Coney Island reconfigured the dizzying effects of urbanism, modernity and the capitalist machine as entertainment, inviting pleasure seekers to experience the shock of modernity as fun. Mechanical amusements celebrated and fostered thrill seekers as sensuous beings who experienced leisure not just through their eyes but with and through their entire bodies. Though the impossibilities of recreating the sensorial experiences of pleasure seekers at Coney Island remains a methodological limitation, this article contributes to literature that understands the senses as lived, embodied phenomena that are products of culture.

A turn-of-the-twentieth century Manhattanite may, perhaps after a long week of working in a factory, have gone on a journey. Boarding a train or a steam-powered boat or a trolley (any of them providing a fairly new experience) she could be transported to the beachside resort of Coney Island. She may have smelled the salt air before she arrived, the anticipation of a day of frolic and relaxation producing a tingling along the surface of her skin and a pleasurable knot in the pit of her stomach. Once disembarked from whatever mode of transportation she had chosen she was free to roam: to walk the beach and see and taste and smell and feel the sea, to wander through the miles of amusements – games of chance, dancing halls, mechanical rides, side shows – the bright lights, the cacophony of barkers and brass bands, the smell of beer and peanuts assaulting her senses. She may have felt hungry and settled at a beachside cafe or an upscale hotel for a cup of clam chowder and a cool drink, the roar of the ocean and the din of the amusement parks rushing over her like waves. She may have decided to splurge a hard-earned dime and enter one of the enclosed amusement parks where she would have been met with unimaginable displays of electric illumination, architectural wonder and technological thrills. She may have decided to get on a mechanical amusement ride, her shrieks of fear and pleasure ringing through the air as she lost her balance and fell into the arms of a fellow rider. Perhaps his hand lingered on her waist for a brief moment until she regained her composure. She may have exited the ride, her senses heightened, face flushed, breath short and decided to return to the beach, to feel the warm sand against her palms and the hot sun on her face, the burst of tiny stars behind her closed eyes like the electric lights that would greet her as the sun set and she boarded train or boat or trolley for her journey back to the city.

This narrative of a fictional pleasure seeker is, of course, conjecture. There is a certain impossibility in reconstructing the sensorial experiences of past subjects, though recent scholarship on the history of the senses has begun doing precisely that.[1] In his article "Making Sense of Social History," Smith locates some of the conundrums surrounding attempts to historicize through sensorial knowledge:

> Should the historian of smell or sound try to actually recreate or experience the odors and noises of the past? Is it actually possible to do so and, if so, is it also desirable? In short, can we really smell and hear (let alone touch, taste and see) the past or are we more limited in what we can achieve? (2003)

Contributing to the difficulties in recreating senses in the past is the concept that the senses are historically located. The way a turn-of-the-twentieth-century pleasure seeker heard the grind of a mechanical amusement and what those sounds signified at that time may be different from one's experience of similar phenomena now. Just as our contemporary experiences of senses are mediated so were those of past subjects, which brings into question the very possibility of knowing the meaning of particular sensorial experiences in the past. We face difficulty, then, in understanding contemporaneously what displays of electric illumination in popular amusement settings may have looked like – and in turn felt like – to the pleasure seekers who experienced them.

The purpose of beginning this article with a fictional figure is to foreground the importance of attempting to do the impossible despite such limitations: to think through sensorial experience as a mediator for social knowledge, both the ways in which contemporary subjects experience their world and the ways in which scholars attempt to theorize the past. To borrow Howes' simple but provocative play on words, studying the senses "makes sense of the past" (2005: 400). One of the assumptions of this essay, and of much of the literature that theorizes and historicizes the sensorium, is that the senses are lived and, quite literally, embodied phenomena that are products of culture (Howes 2005: 3). This opens a space for understanding the senses as historically situated and culturally specific. It would be incorrect to claim, for instance, that sensorial experience is a "modern" phenomenon: humans have always experienced the world through their senses. What I aim to explore, however, is the ways in which Coney Island's enclosed amusement parks capitalized on sensorial experience and escalated it to monumental proportions, transformed spectacle as total-body sensations and invited thrill seekers to experience amusement with and through their entire bodies.

Coney Island at the turn of the twentieth century provided urbanite thrill seekers with an inundation of sensorial overload. Walking through the gates at Coney Island's three enclosed amusement parks (Steeplechase, 1897, Luna Park, 1903 and Dreamland, 1904) catapulted thrill seekers into dreams of phantasmagoria: a "blend of machine technologies and art galleries, military cannons and fashion costumes, business and pleasure, synthesized into one dazzling visual experience" (Buck-Morss 1989: 5). The juxtaposition of spectacular displays of technology with sensorial overload forced modern subjects to forge new relationships to the ways that they consumed and experienced entertainment. The kinesthetic thrill of mechanical rides, amusement park exhibits and architecture and the location of Coney Island on the beachside in close proximity to the metropolis blended to produce spectacle that was increasingly not solely about *seeing* but about *feeling*. The consumption of mass culture was bound up in corporeal experience that radically transformed pleasure seekers' relationship to their bodies and to the bodies of others in the public sphere. While the transformation of spectacle as corporeal would reach its epoch in the enclosed amusement park era, as to be examined shortly, accounts of Coney Island's Sodom by the Sea era highlight the sensorial pleasures to be found at the amusement resort.

**Coney Island: A Sodom by the Sea**
Throughout its development as a beachside resort, Coney Island reconfigured how pleasure seekers sought to spend their leisure time and expendable income. Coney Island borrowed the innovations of urban popular amusements and placed them within a seemingly ideal location: the beachside. Coney Island's close proximity to Manhattan and its natural amenities made it a popular beachside resort for Manhattanites seeking refuge from the growing metropolis. With its unspoiled natural landscape, the island provided a back-to-nature getaway from the metropolis – what Rem Koolhaas characterized as "a factory of man-made experience, where the real and the natural ceased to exist" – that allowed for the sensuous consumption of nature and the sensorial experience of entertainment (1994: 10).

In the 1820s a direct road and the island's first hotel were erected, thereby inaugurating Coney Island as an easily accessible respite from the growing metropolis for those with their own transportation.[2] Multifarious forms of public transportation soon followed and a transportation boom emerged and peaked from the mid 1860s to the early 1890s providing several transportation options for beach-bound patrons. As Weinstein (1984: 92) makes clear, "Coney Island's leap from obscurity to the forefront of beach resorts in the world would not have been possible without easily accessible, moderately priced transportation." The proliferation of public transportation to Coney Island aided in its success but was also a source of ambivalence: as print materials in the last quarter of the nineteenth century indicate, the "publicness" implicit in public transportation meant that anyone with the monetary means could use it, and as the *Atlantic Monthly* succinctly put it in 1874, Coney Island was "unfashionable" "since its advantages are attainable by all" (Shanley 1874: 306). With the advent of public transportation to its shores, Coney Island, which was outside the New York City and Brooklyn police jurisdictions, was increasingly frequented by "undesirables" – characterized during the period as gamblers, prostitutes and con artists. Advances in public transportation helped transform the character of the island from a peaceful, uninhabited beachside paradise to a Sodom by the Sea.[3]

The West End of Coney Island became infamous – or, at the very least, was vilified in print – for illicit and immoral behavior, behavior that was interestingly associated with corporeality and the senses. A *Harper's Weekly* article (Mines 1891) describes the West End of Coney Island as a cacophony of sounds and sensorial overloads, "a most extraordinary jumble" where "conflicting strains of music came from everywhere." Amusements to be found at the West End, it noted, included: "[re]volving swings and merry-go-rounds, shooting galleries and concert halls, razzle-dazzles and switch-backs, toboggan rollers and photographers. Frankfurters and pea-nuts, beer, music, noise" (ibid.). Many of the items listed were quotidian objects that thrill seekers would have access to such as beer and music. Their juxtaposition with more spectacular and constructed environments such as concert halls and merry-go-rounds creates a defamiliarization of everyday objects, thereby reconfiguring the quotidian as strange and appeals to the senses as noteworthy at Coney Island's West End.

The combination and intensification of the senses at the West End continued to receive attention from the press as emblematic of Coney's purported moral decline. An *Atlantic Monthly* article from 1874 (Shanley: 309) depicts the West End as a "lunatic asylum" and suggests that even "reputable" folks became transformed by the chaos and disorder that overtakes them once they set foot on that part of the beach. Coney's transformative powers oscillated around the pleasure seekers' abandonment of restraint and such abandonment was often depicted as succumbing to one's senses. Those visiting the West End become "inmates" of the lunatic asylum, loosing any semblance of morality or culture they may have had as they allow themselves to become overwhelmed by their physical experiences. "The women flap around and about in the water and scream like the fowls to which that element is natural" while "[n]umbers of the men lie wallowing for hours in the sand, in which they roll like wild beasts, rubbing it madly into their hair and plastering themselves all over with it" (Shanley 1874: 309). In this depiction, visitors become animalistic and primitive as the sensorial overload of the West End takes over their rational faculties. The carnivalesque atmosphere of the West End was blamed for transforming pleasure seekers into uncontrolled (and uncontrollable) primitive beings. These critiques make evident that pleasure seekers were forging new relationships with morally acceptable behavior in the public sphere, the concept of leisure time and activity and their bodies as sensorial beings.

Pleasure seekers learned that Coney Island was not sedentary and passive but was to be experienced with the entire body and all the senses. The sensorial experience of Coney Island was clearly a point of contestation – evidenced in the moniker "Sodom by the Sea" and in critiques outlined above – but experiencing spectacle as all sensorial continued (and escalated) when three monumental amusement parks opened in rapid succession around the turn of the twentieth century and placed Coney Island in the center of the amusement world.

## Coney Island's Enclosed Amusement Park Era: Fantasy Lands and the Shock of Modernity

In 1897, George Tilyou opened Steeplechase Park, the first major and longest lasting amusement park at Coney Island. By building a fence around an entertainment area and charging an admission fee, producers were able to control the ethos of the parks by dictating the amusements that were located in them and spectators that were allowed to visit them. By enclosing amusement parks, their originators were creating contained, hermetically-sealed spaces that could fabricate and control the ethos of the park. By excluding illegal activities and those characters of purported ill repute the enclosed amusement parks at Coney Island became locations of respectable, clean entertainment.

Coney Island's second major amusement park, Luna Park (1903), was predicated on taking spectators out of their everyday, urban experience and transporting them to another world. Tilyou, who saw the "Trip to the Moon" exhibit at the Pan-American Exposition of 1901, invited the creators of the exhibit, Frederic Thompson and Elmer (Skip) Dundy, to move it to Steeplechase Park. After a successful season in 1902, Thompson and Dundy decided to construct their own amusement park at Coney Island, topically and architecturally conceived around the concept of an out-of-this-world fantasy land. The architecture, rides and exhibits at Luna Park were meant to be specimens of the moon: patrons would leave their quotidian preoccupations at the gates and enter another world. Thompson aimed to fabricate spectators' experience on every level and believed that "the spirit of gaiety and emotional excitement in a park must be manufactured – via scenery, lights, shows, and buildings ... an 'other word,' a fantastic fairy land or dream city, must be created" (Weinstein 1984: 132). Since Luna Park's innovative use of design to create another world the construction of a dream world has become the benchmark of amusement parks (Weinstein 1984: 132).

Luna Park constructed a space that visually embodied the future and represented progress. Thompson claimed that the success of Luna Park depended on its ability to change continuously: "'You see, this being the moon, it is always changing ... A stationary Luna Park would be an anomaly'" (quoted in Koolhaas 1994: 41). Executing his theory that progress is predicated on this continual cycle of creation and destruction, Thompson radically reconstructed Luna Park every new season.[4] "The equation of Luna Park with 'lunar change,'" argues Register (2001: 121), "provided a rich synthesis of the way the resort combined artifice with nature, the quest for novelty with premodern myth, systematic managed technology with the improprieties of carnivalesque dreams of plenty." By engineering constantly reimagined displays of spectacle, Luna Park mirrored – albeit in a more spectacular and fabricated way – the constantly changing urban order. The invitation to enter this fantasy land was an invitation to spectators to become corporeally engaged in the manufacture and consumption of spectacle, spectacle that was not solely visual but that appealed to all of the senses.

Across the way from Luna Park's spectacular dream world, Dreamland opened its doors in 1904 with its own version of the enclosed amusement park. Though Dreamland replicated many of the innovations developed at its predecessors, Steeplechase and Luna Park, it explicitly divorced itself from the prior two amusement parks. While Steeplechase boasted inexpensive prices that could be afforded by all and Luna Park heralded its cacophony of sounds, sights and architectural wonders, Dreamland advertised itself as clean, spacious and devoid of chaos. Conceived by politician and realtor William H. Reynolds, who wanted to build a "higher class" amusement park, Dreamland was designed to be the antithesis of New York City's noise, crowds and congestion. Reynolds employed many of the design principles he used to create the suburban community of Borough Park, an area with detached private homes and wide streets that catered to the upwardly-mobile middle class. Influenced by the architecture of world fairs and turn-of-the-century urban planning movements, Dreamland was designed as a more genteel amusement park meant to appeal to a "higher" class of patrons.

At the safe, homogeneous White City, Dreamland discursively and aesthetically equated whiteness with purity and with wealth. The construction of a safe, clean Dreamland was consolidated in its aesthetic sensibilities and referenced the "White City" at the Chicago World's Columbian Exposition of 1893. Both Dreamland and the Chicago Exposition constructed utopian White Cities that symbolized purity and the purging of contaminating elements. According to Rydell, the White City at the Chicago Exposition was a "manifestation of what was good in American life" and served not only as a dream-like getaway but also as a didactic model of how America and Americans, should be (1984: 40). Similarly, the White City at Dreamland sought to illustrate bourgeois sensibilities and instruct the middle- and working-class about proper, clean, respectable entertainment. Dreamland's innovative brand may have also been its failure: the park never achieved the success of the other amusement parks. While theories of Dreamland's failure abound, it is provocative to imagine that Dreamland's attempts to create order was antithetical to the very ethos of Coney Island as experiential leisure that appealed to all of the senses. While thrill seekers may have wanted a respite from the chaos of the metropolis, they may not quite have been looking for the clean, orderly, suburban getaway that Dreamland promised.

Though the three major enclosed amusement parks had different aesthetic sensibilities and ideological objectives, by the turn of the twentieth century, Coney Island provided the best that modernism and nature had to offer. The island had become a beacon of technological innovation that reconfigured the consumption of leisure as participatory and kinesthetic. Spectacle became not solely a visual experience but a corporeal one, an experience that catapulted pleasure seekers out of their everyday experiences into unexpected and fantastic circumstances. As Immerso (2002: 87) puts it, the "melding of ornamentation and centrifugal force gave the Coney Island amusement park its extraordinary dynamism."

Part of the thrill of the amusement park was the continual exposure to new stimuli, those tiny jolts of the unexpected that shocked the senses. Buck-Morss locates shock within amusement parks and, with help from Walter Benjamin, defines it as constitutive of modernity:

> In industrial production no less than modern warfare, in street crowds and erotic encounters, in amusement parks and gambling casinos, shock is the very essence of modern experience. The technologically altered environment exposes the human sensorium to physical shocks that have their correspondence in psychic shock. (Buck-Morss 1992)

For Benjamin (1983: 116), shock had become the "norm" of modern life.[5] In his reading of Baudelaire, Benjamin (1968: 175) shows the close relationship between shock and the metropolitan masses, the way an urbanite would plunge "into the crowd as into a reservoir of electric energy." Coping with the shock of the city streets was further exacerbated by new technologies that "subjected the human sensorium to a complex kind of training" (ibid.). Coney Island's enclosed amusement parks – with their physically jarring mechanical rides, exploitation of technological innovation to shock and wow spectators and their crowded environments that both mirrored and deflected the metropolitan street – helped to usher in what Benjamin argues had, by the 1920s, become the norm and a marker of modern life: shock (Benjamin1983: 116). Benjamin laments that "the disintegration of the aura in the experience of shock" was the price paid by and for the modern era. But the shock at Coney Island was of a different order. Rather than disintegrative, shock at Coney Island was reconfigured as rejuvenating, as part and parcel of a new experience of leisure as participatory and kinesthetic (Benjamin 1968: 194).

## The Thrill of the Ride: Mechanical Amusements, Kineticism and Capitalism

The shock that became the marker of the modern era had a literal manifestation in the physical jolts of mechanical rides. With their celebration of speed and kineticism, mechanical amusements consolidated many of the innovations of the modern era from the electric illumination that lit up the rides to the science of centrifugal force that propelled bodies through space. The kinesthetic thrill of mechanical amusements was bound up in their recreation of dangerous situations. As Rabinovitz (2001) points out, mechanical attractions "were simulations of danger; they provided a tenuous relationship between the perception of danger and the assurance of safety." Part of the thrill of amusement rides and exhibits and spectators' eagerness to place themselves in situations that were possibly dangerous outside of the context of the amusement park, was a momentary suspension of control. Pleasure seekers were fascinated with, as Rabinovitz (ibid.: 90) claimed, the "imagination of disaster, the fantasy of seeing technology go out of control." The setting of the amusement park allowed spectators to experience the fear of chaos in a controlled setting. By preserving the excitement while expelling any real danger, Coney Island's mechanical rides and staged exhibits presented pleasure seekers with images and experiences that were thrilling yet benign.

Another part of the thrill of mechanical amusements was surrendering one's body to the machine and to technology. Physical contact initiated from mechanical amusements was not necessarily considered to be a product of the individual's agency. Rapid-motion mechanical rides had explicitly sexual overtones: couples (or complete strangers!) were thrown together from the movement of the rides and girls' skirts would fly suggestively above their ankles. Though extremely tame to a contemporary audience, such explicit physical contact and public displays of the body marked a radical shift away from conservative, Victorian-age sensibilities about what was considered morally acceptable behavior in the public sphere. As their behavior was a product of a "machine," and therefore circumvented by the undeniable progress thought to be inherent to science, couples were not consciously embracing in an unrestrained display of immoral behavior. Mechanical amusements allowed spectators to behave in a slightly out of control manner in an ultimately controlled setting. While providing a sensorial overload to thrill seekers, mechanical amusements also transformed what was considered morally acceptable behavior in the public sphere.

Mechanical amusements invited pleasure seekers to experience the markers of capitalism with all of their senses, a process that allowed for the reconfiguration of what Marx located as the desensitizing of subjects under industrialization. According to Marx, the alienation of the senses under capitalism affected all segments of the population: the proletariat became deprived of sensorial stimulation while the bourgeoisie forwent sensuous pleasures as their senses were "ultimately fixed on one object – capital" (Howes, 2005: 282–3). Factories forced workers to "keep up with the machine," eliminating any creative, non-mechanical processes that may clog the flow of the system. In the factory, there was little opportunity for sensorial experience; in fact it was felt that workers might perform better when desensitized. As Buck-Morss (1995) explains,

> the factory system injures every one of the human senses, paralyzing the imagination of the worker. His or her work is "sealed off from experience"; memory is replaced by conditioned response, learning by "drill," skill by repetition: "practice counts for nothing."

One of the results of capitalism and industrialization, according to Marx and others, is that the worker becomes cut off from his senses. To put it another way, workers are forced to become mechanical, to become like machines themselves. Marx laments this transformation for it denies the fact that humans are living beings and part of one's humanity is to be a being that senses: "To be sensuous, i.e. to be real, is to be an object of sense, a sensuous object, thus to have sensuous objects outside oneself, to have objects of sense perception" (1977:104). The tedium of factory work obliterates humans' sense perceptions and thus their "realness" as "sensuous" beings – a precondition for their very humanity according to Marx – is denied.

Mechanical amusement rides at Coney Island to a certain degree reversed some of the negative effects of the desensitizing of the factory and the capitalist machine. Though pleasure seekers were not technically in control of machines of pleasure, they willingly placed themselves in the position of objects of mechanization. Unlike the factory worker whose senses were cut off from them as they were forced to become machine-like in their labor, mechanical amusements heightened the modern subjects' senses. Mechanical amusements brilliantly invoked the very markers of industrial capitalism – mechanization, standardization, the giving of the body to the machine – while inverting the power structure inherent in such a system to reconfigure pleasure seekers' experience of both industrialization and leisure. The endless cycle of tedious factory work was momentarily suspended with mechanical amusements that escalated the senses. Pleasure seekers laughed, they screamed, they cried – often in rapid succession and seemingly simultaneously. Their senses were altered and heightened through mechanical technology, a first cousin to the very industrialization that had severed their senses in the first place. Pleasure seekers choose to be out of control; they choose to have their bodies catapulted through space in highly controlled though unexpected ways. In other words, they knew that something would happen, but they could not predict, nor could they replicate, their experience of the ride. Mechanical amusements produced lived, in the moment experiences and, in turn, sensuous beings, a precondition for one's humanity.

## Spectacle as Total Body Experience: Sensorial Consumption

As a phenomenon of the post-industrial revolution, amusement parks mark the shift in American culture from "an economy based on labor and production to one dominated by patterns of consumption and leisure" (Weinstein 1984: 143). Such patterns of consumption and leisure were epitomized in the popularization of department stores, museums, public parks, world's fairs and amusement parks, to name but a few possibilities. Consumer culture's construction of spectators as consumers had profound impacts not only on the types of leisure activities available to and partaken by pleasure seekers but also on their relationship to the public sphere and visuality. Such visuality was not simply about seeing: the new consumer culture heralded being seen.[6]

Pleasure seekers could enter these fantasy worlds at a price, both economically and ideologically. The ideological price paid in such a "dream world" of mass consumption constructed buyers as mass consumers (Williams 1982). As Rosalind Williams shows (1982: 58–106), the late nineteenth century marked a transition in culture to the sensual pleasure of consumption. The sensuality of consumer culture was bound up in not only looking at but touching objects for sale. The department stores that emerged reconfigured consumers' relationship to commodities. By placing fixed prices on items and allowing consumers the pleasure of browsing, the department store created a fantasy world of commodities that facilitated new relationships to buying. While with mercantile capitalism consumers would bargain with shop owners and might, to some degree, feel committed to purchasing a negotiated item, department stores allowed for consumer autonomy as one could browse and touch objects for sale without feeling any commitment to buy. Howes (2005: 284) argues that the "sensory stimulation" of the department store seduced buyers with its "theatrical lighting, enticing window displays and its floor after floor of enticing merchandise." Department stores became dream worlds that displayed commodities in an increasingly participatory way as browsing and touching became part of the process of consuming. Similarly, the sensual pleasure of consumption at the enclosed amusement parks at Coney Island was bound up with thrill seeking that was increasingly participatory and kinesthetic.

Upon walking through the gates at one of the enclosed amusement parks at Coney Island, thrill seekers were inundated with a cacophony of sounds, sights, smells and sensations that, quite literally, overwhelmed the senses. To fully experience the thrill of Coney Island required that new relationships be forged between spectators' bodies, the bodies of others and the new technologies that participated in and facilitated this transformation in the first place. As Rabinovitz makes clear, Coney Island's amusement parks helped to "define a new concept of urban modernism – the celebration of kineticism and speed, the beauty of industrial technologies, and the experience of the crowd"(2001: 85). The sensorial overload experienced at Coney Island's enclosed amusement parks – the bombardment and exaggeration of sight, sound and kinesthesia – helped constitute the modern subject by unifying the "fragmentary nature of urban experience through a new type of leisure" (ibid.). This new modern subject *experienced* leisure activities in different ways than their preceding generations.

At Coney Island's amusement parks, spectators increasingly came to experience the rides and exhibits with their entire bodies. Spectacle became not simply about seeing but also about feeling and experiencing. To fully experience the spectacle at Coney Island's enclosed amusement parks necessitated a transformation in spectators' relationship to their senses. Pleasure seekers needed to integrate their senses to process the sensorial overload provided by the kinesthetic thrills of the amusement park. As Kasson (1978: 49) rightfully acknowledges, "photographs give some indication of this [environmental phantasmagoria], but they alone cannot do it justice." Instead he invites the reader to envision the total-body experience of pleasure seekers at Coney Island:

> We must try to imagine the smells of circus animals, the taste of hot dogs, beer and seafood, the jostle of surrounding revelers, the speed and jolts of amusement rides, and, what especially impressed observers, the din of barkers, brass bands, roller coasters, merry-go-rounds, shooting galleries ... above all, the shouts and laughter of the crowd itself. (ibid.)

The introduction to this article pays homage to Kasson's methodological quest by fictionalizing a pleasure seeker's sensorial experience of Coney Island. While Kasson focuses on the historian attempting to understand Coney Island, we should also pay particular attention to thinking through the spectators' experience of this sensorial overload in the service of attempting to contextualize the senses in a modern, urban, industrial order. The modern subject who made sense of this phantasmagoria was not solely an "I" with an "eye" but was an integrated, total body with complex sense perceptions. The kinesthetic excitement produced from mechanical amusements and exhibits at Coney Island amusement parks reconfigured spectacle as a total body experience.

The island's invitation to experience leisure kinesthetically exemplified a larger transformation in modern subjects' relationship to visuality and the senses. As scholars have made evident, the "senses are typically ordered in hierarchies" (Howes 2005: 10). The valorization of vision during the Enlightenment period was connected to the establishment of dominant political, social and aesthetic regimes (Jay 1993: 49). Touch and smell were devaluated as they were considered "more intimate" and thereby less reliable than vision (ibid.). Related to the equation of intimacy and the unreliability of particular senses, Classen shows how the lower senses of touch, taste and smell were attributed to women – and thereby configured as "feminine in nature" – while men had "mastery of the 'higher' senses" (2005: 70). The devaluation of the non-visual senses and the valorization of vision were considered to be part of the "civilizing process" according to Martin Jay (1993: 49). Modernism disrupted the Enlightenment's avowal of the link between light and rationality and claims of sight as the most noble and hearing as the least reliable of the senses (ibid.: 85).

It is important to note that the senses, though they have been conceived of as hierarchical and gendered, are socially located but not static. The experience of going to the beach at Coney Island was multisensory: feeling the crashing waves against your body and the hot sand in your fingers; smelling clam chowder and the salty ocean; hearing music and shrieks of pleasure-terror from the shock of cool water and patrons on mechanical rides; tasting cold beer and roasted peanuts; seeing unimaginable displays of electric illumination. Many of these experiences appealed to multiple senses simultaneously. The ocean was not simply to be seen but was to be pleasurably experienced with all the senses: the salt could be tasted, the warm sand and cool water could be felt, the crashing waves could be heard. Though this multi-sensory experience of phenomena is not necessarily particular to Coney Island's beach – almost all beaches are experienced in this way – the man made and the natural sensorial overload of Coney Island invited spectators to experience the amusement parks with their entire bodies. Coney Island transformed the hierarchy of the senses, both in terms of gender division and in terms of the valorization of particular senses over others, by inviting pleasure seekers to do that from which they had been dissuaded in the past: to recognize, to revel in and to celebrate themselves as sensorial beings.

Producers offered up new attractions to a public disenchanted with exhibits that only engaged vision and offered modern pleasure seekers amusements that appealed to the sensorium. Explicitly referencing this transformation from spectacle as solely visual to spectacle as all-sensory, one of the creators of Luna Park, Fred Thompson, acknowledged the new consumer who "was no longer satisfied solely by the 'appeal to the eye.' Now ... the customer demanded to 'hear the boat crash or the train fall apart' or to feel 'the sensation of going down some dizzy incline'" (Register 2001: 118). Thompson responded to and helped perpetuate this reconfiguration of spectacle as all sensorial by creating exhibits that spectators could feel, smell, hear and even taste. As pleasure seekers became increasingly interested in encountering entertainment corporally, exhibitors responded with amusement rides and exhibits that demanded spectators engage all of their senses. Entertainment became not solely a passive, visual exploit but an event to be experienced through their bodies.

Thompson's acknowledgement of the new consumer's desire to be entertained corporeally locates a larger shift in what Crary has shown as the transformation in the subject's relationship to visuality in the nineteenth century. In *Techniques of the Observer*, Crary demonstrates a "'liberation of vision" in the 1820s and 1830s that transformed subjects into observers and locates this transformation as "a product of and at the same time constitutive of modernity" (ibid.: 9). By locating this new subject within the context of "modernity," Crary argues (ibid. 11) that modernity is in fact inseparable from "a remaking of the observer." New scopic regimes and new industrial techniques reposition the observer "into an undemarcated terrain on which the distinction between internal sensation and external signs is irrevocably blurred" (ibid.: 24). This repositioning destabilizes vision as simply and solely representational; Crary persuasively shows that vision comes to be located in the observer's body, thereby making observation "increasingly a question of equivalent sensations and stimuli." (ibid.).

## Conclusion

Coney Island's enclosed amusement parks escalated observation as sensation, particularly in its mechanical amusements that celebrated kineticism, speed and the machine and blurred the distinction between one's senses and external stimuli. Coney Island was both emblematic of and contributed to this larger remaking of the observer, according to Crary, the desensitization of the factory worker, according to Marx and the shock of modernism, according to Benjamin. What made Coney Island unique was that it explicitly staged the markers of modernism, urbanism and industrialization within a context of sensorial entertainment. Coney Island made the newness of the modern era fun: the machine that was emblematic of the industrial age and the shock of modernity were reconstituted as pleasurable. Part and parcel of this pleasure, of all this fun, was the invitation for it to be, the expectation that it would be, experienced with one's entire being.

Our fictional pleasure seeker at the beginning of this article did precisely that: she experienced the enclosed amusement parks and Coney Island's beach with her entire body. For her, travel and leisure were bound up with sensorial experience and corporeality. I would like to suggest that, though she is fictional, I do not believe her experience is necessarily a fiction. What I mean to foreground in such a claim is that methodological limitations should not hinder our attempts to think about or theorize the important role that the senses have played in mediating people's experiences and even in our understanding of the past. To understand the thrill and attraction of Coney Island at the turn of the twentieth century requires us to think through what was unique about it. The feature that stands out, the ontology of Coney Island if you will, was its carnivalesque atmosphere, the constant bombardment of sites and sounds and smells that, quite literally, overwhelmed the senses. I must concede that I will never be able to recreate, nor could I comprehend, a pleasure seeker's first experience of a mechanical amusement ride or unimaginable displays of electric illumination. Though there is a certain impossibility in reconstructing the sensorial experience of such past subjects this article seeks to do the impossible: to trace and theorize the ways that Coney Island helped transform spectacle into a sensorial experience.

## Notes
1. See, for example, readers such Harvey 2003, Bull and Back 2003 and David Howes 2005 (particularly Howes' Introduction and the conclusion, which outline scholarship on the senses and a bibliography of sensory research). The former two titles are part of Berg's provocative "Sensory Formations" series that is dedicated to publishing literature on the senses.
2. The Coney Island Causeway was built in 1824. The opening of the Coney Island Hotel is often dated at 1829, though Weinstein (1984: 47 fn. 45) claims the hotel opened in 1824.
3. For an extended discussion of this term and an early history of Coney Island, see Pilot and Ranson 1941.
4. For a detailed list of seasonal changes at Coney Island, see Stanton 2005.
5. See also Benjamin 1968, particularly the chapter "On Some Motifs in Baudelaire."
6. In *The Birth of the Museum* (Bennett 1995), Tony Bennett puts forth the concept of the exhibitionary complex to understand the new emerging mass culture's mode of organizing power through display that was predicated not only on seeing but being seen.

## References
Benjamin, Walter. 1968. *Illuminations.* Trans. Harry Zohn. New York: Schocken Books.
———. 1983. *Charles Baudelaire.* Trans. Harry Zohn. London: Verso.
Bennett, Tony. 1995. *The Birth of the Museum: History, Theory, Politics.* London: Routledge.
Buck-Morss, Susan. 1989. *The Dialectics of Seeing: Walter Benjamin and the Arcades Project.* Cambridge, MA: MIT Press.

——. 1992. "Aesthetics and Anaesthetics: Walter Benjamin's Artwork Essay Reconsidered." *October*, Autumn, 62: 3–41.

——. 1995. "The City as Dreamworld and Catastrophe." *October*, Summer, 73: 3–26.

Bull, Michael and Les Back (eds). 2003. *The Auditory Culture Reader.* Oxford: Berg.

Classen, Constance. 2005."The Witch's Senses: Sensory Ideologies and Transgressive Femininities from the Renaissance to Modernity." In David Howes (ed.), *Empire of The Senses.* Oxford, UK: Berg.

Crary, Jonathan. 1990. *Techniques of the Observer: On Vision and Modernity in the Nineteenth Century.* Cambridge, MA: MIT Press.

Harvey, Elizabeth D. (ed.). 2003. *Sensible Flesh: On Touch in Early Modern Culture.* Philadelphia: University of Pennsylvania Press.

Howes, David (ed.). 2005. *Empire of the Senses: The Sensual Culture Reader.* Oxford: Berg.

Howes, David. 2005. "Hyperesthesia, or, The Sensual Logic of Late Capitalism." In David Howes (ed.), *Empire of The Senses.* Oxford: Berg.

Immerso, Michael. 2002. *Coney Island: The People's Playground.* New Brunswick: Rutgers University Press.

Jay, Martin. 1993. *Downcast Eyes: The Denigration of Vision in Twentieth-Century French Thought.* Berkeley: University of California Press.

Kasson, John F. 1978. *Amusing the Million: Coney Island at the Turn of the Century.* New York: Hill & Wang.

Koolhaas, Rem. 1994. *Delirious New York.* New York: Montacelli Press.

Mines, Flavel Scott. 1891. "A Pilgrimage to Coney Island." *Harper's Weekly* (September 12), 694–5.

Pilot, Oliver and Ranson, Jo. 1941. *Sodom by the Sea: An Affectionate History of Coney Island*. New York: Doubleday.

Rabinovitz, Lauren. 2001. "Urban Wonderlands: Siting Modernity in Turn-of-the-Century Amusement Parks." *European Contributions to American Studies*, 45(1): 85–97.

Register, Woody. 2001. *The Kid of Coney Island: Fred Thompson and the Rise of American Amusements.* Oxford: Oxford University Press.

Rydell, Robert. 1984. *All the World's a Fair.* Chicago: University of Chicago Press.

Shanley, Charles Dawson. 1874. "Coney Island." *Atlantic Monthly* (September), 306–12.

Smith, Mark M. 2003. "Making Sense of Social History." *Journal of Social History*, 37(1): 165–86.

Stanton, Jeffrey. 2005 [2003]. *"Coney Island."* Available online: http://naid.sppsr.ucla.edu/coneyisland/.

Weinstein, Stephen. 1984. "The Nickel Empire: Coney Island and the Creation of Urban Seaside Resorts in the United States." Ph.D. thesis, Columbia University, New York.

Williams, Rosalind H. 1982. *Dream Worlds: Mass Consumption in Late Nineteenth-Century France.* Berkeley: University of California Press.

# JOURNAL OF THE
## SOCIETY FOR VISUAL ANTHROPOLOGY

# Visual Anthropology Review

**A**s the journal of the Society for Visual Anthropology, *Visual Anthropology Review* promotes the discussion of visual studies, broadly conceived. Within its breadth, visual anthropology includes both the study of visual aspects of human behavior and the use of visual media in anthropological research, representation and teaching. The journal welcomes articles, reviews and commentary on the use of multimedia, still photography, film, video and non-camera generated images, as well as on visual ideologies, indigenous media, applied visual anthropology, art, dance, gesture, sign language, human movement, museology, architecture and material culture.

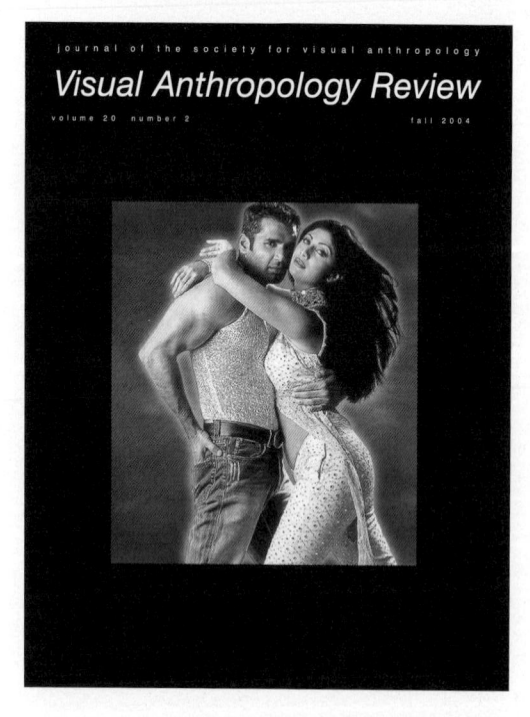

Visual Anthropology Review
http://etext.virginia.edu/VAR/

# The Sensory Dimensions of Gardening

## Christopher Tilley

Christopher Tilley is Professor of Material Culture in the Dept of Anthropology, University College London. Recent books include *The Materiality of Stone: Explorations in Landscape Phenomenology* (2004), *Metaphor and Material Culture* (1999) and *An Ethnography of the Neolithic* (1996).
c.tilley@ucl.ac.uk

ABSTRACT This paper considers the multiple sensory dimensions of gardening and their synesthetic significance in an ethnographic study of gardens and gardening in England and Sweden. It challenges the notion that the different senses (vision, smell, sound, touch and taste) can be considered in hierarchical terms i.e. some as being more important than others in an assessment of the meaning and significance of gardening as an everyday practice. It argues that there is a significant difference between what people say and what they actually do and that when we study the latter the significance of all the senses in relation to each other is highlighted.

An important development in material culture studies in recent years has been the growing realization of the significance of the multisensorial qualities of artifacts as a key to understanding their meaning and significance. The various sensory qualities that artifacts possess – the look, the feel and weight, the sound, the odor and taste of things, and the sensory skills and values that are part and parcel of their production, exchange and consumption have come to the forefront of analysis in a number of recent discussions of material culture (e.g. Buchli 2002; Bull and Back 2003; Tilley 2001; 2004; Howes 2005; Classen 2005; Tilley et al . 2006), so much so that Howes refers to this as a "sensory revolution" (Howes 2005; 2006: 161) whose critical counterpoint is the excesses of the metaphor of the text in the contemporary social sciences. The manner in which we sense material forms has become as crucial to discuss as the way in which they might be "read" or "written." Taking on board the differing sensorial dimensions of things allows us to appreciate more fully the thickly constituted and multidimensional phenomenological experiences of artifacts, with which we always engage with the full range of our human senses, and the manner in which the things themselves become of such significance to our lives that they actively mediate how think and how we act.

A garden is of particular interest to study ethnographically in this respect because, unlike virtually any other artifact in contemporary Western culture, it is *commonly* acknowledged to have multidimensional sensorial qualities that overlap and are intertwined and affect the gardener. Thus gardeners will ordinarily remark, in everyday conversation, about visual domains of experience, e.g. the color and appearance of the garden, acoustic domains of experience such as bird song or the sound of falling rain, the olfactory domains of experience – the scent of flowers or of newly mown grass – tactile domains of experience such as the feel of smooth bark or a well-used tool in their hands and the taste of fruit and vegetables they have grown themselves that can never be matched by the most magnificent one might buy in a shop. For most of the time appreciating the garden is thus a synesthetic experience involving all the five human senses – sight, smell, touch, sound and taste, which usually intermingle and feed into each other.

Generally, the range and depth and personal and cultural significance of this sensory interaction between the gardener and the garden is unremarkable. It therefore goes largely undiscussed and unacknowledged. The argument of this paper is that it in fact constitutes one of the primary reasons why so many people find gardening such a deeply rewarding and satisfying emotional experience. These manifold sensory perceptions of the garden form a fundamental part of the emotions that creating and working in the garden generates in the gardener.

Ostensibly, gardening is all about cultivating plants. At a much deeper level, I want to suggest, it is actually about cultivating the soul through cultivating the earth. Through the expressive medium of the human body itself, through utilizing and exploring its entire range of sensory and perceptive capacitities, gardening as a craft and as a productive activity, is a primary way of redressing the existential alienation inevitably produced in a culture of mass production and mass consumption. We live without any longer making that which we consume and, for much of the time sit in offices and houses remaining cut off and insulated, suffering varying degrees of sensory deprivation, from the living world beyond.

This ethnographic study is based on extended interviews with, and selected participant observation of, 62 southern Swedish gardeners (27 male and 35 female) and 65 southern English gardeners (26 male and 39 female) conducted during the summer months between 2000 and 2004. In both countries gardening is by far the most popular outdoor leisure pursuit and an activity completely transcending socioeconomic, gender and age differences. The approach taken is multi-sited (Marcus 1995) involving interviews with informants from Malmö in the southwest of Sweden to Stockholm in the northeast, and from Exeter in the west of England to London in the east.

The results discussed here are part of a much wider study of the meaning and significance of gardens and gardening in contemporary Western culture, based on a study of as representative a sample as possible of ordinary domestic and allotment gardens and gardeners in both countries from a wide variety of different socioeconomic backgrounds. For some gardening was their sole or main interest, for others the garden was simply an area of land around the house that they had to cope with, or tend, in some way.

At an early stage in the interviews, which took place in their own gardens, all the gardeners were asked to fill out a simple form ticking which of the sensory dimensions of the garden were very important, important or not important to them (see Tables 1–3). Some time after that, in structured and unstructured questions, their responses were

**Table 1.** The Significance of Different Sensory Dimensions of the Garden According to English Gardeners

| Sensory dimension | Very important N | % | Important N | % | Not important N | % |
|---|---|---|---|---|---|---|
| Vision/appearance | 49 | 75 | 16 | 25 | 0 | 0 |
| Smell/scent | 27 | 42 | 33 | 51 | 5 | 7 |
| Touch/texture | 17 | 26 | 30 | 46 | 18 | 28 |
| Sound | 23 | 36 | 32 | 49 | 10 | 15 |
| Taste | 16 | 25 | 16 | 25 | 33 | 50 |

Number (N) of informants = 65

**Table 2.** The Significance of Different Sensory Dimensions of the Garden According to Swedish Gardeners

| Sensory dimension | Very important N | % | Important N | % | Not important N | % |
|---|---|---|---|---|---|---|
| Vision/appearance | 43 | 69 | 19 | 31 | 0 | 0 |
| Smell/scent | 23 | 37 | 30 | 48 | 9 | 15 |
| Touch/texture | 12 | 20 | 22 | 35 | 28 | 45 |
| Sound | 21 | 34 | 21 | 34 | 20 | 32 |
| Taste | 11 | 18 | 27 | 44 | 24 | 38 |

Number (N) of informants = 62

further explored. Preferring to let people speak as far as possible in their own words, I quote extensively from these responses below. The principal results of the preliminary form filling exercise were remarkably similar for all categories of English and Swedish gardeners and did not differ significantly according to whether they were English or Swedish, what type of garden they had (e.g. large or small, urban, suburban or rural), their occupation and income, degree of knowledge or interest in gardening.

The visual appearance and form of the garden was of overriding significance. No gardeners said this was not important to them whereas all the other sensory dimensions of the garden were unimportant to at least some. Smell, or scent, was ranked as the second most significant sensory dimension with sound being of almost equal importance. Touch was only very important to a quarter of gardeners while taste was regarded as unimportant to half of English gardeners and 38 percent of Swedish gardeners.

Vision and smell in the garden were always unproblematic categories that did not require any further explanation. However, touch, sound and taste did need explication for many. Before filling out the form many gardeners asked what I meant by touch, sound and taste in the garden. It was not, of course, that they had not experienced these sensory dimensions of being in the garden, more that they just had not consciously thought about them, and especially not as separate categories of experience. When I explained to them that by touch I was referring to how the plants felt (e.g. smooth or spiky, glossy or rough) or things such as the differing textures of tree bark, stone or soil, by sound, such things as bird song or traffic noise or the noise of lawnmowers, and by taste, the taste of fruit and vegetables then these also became easily recognizable sensory dimensions of the garden to them. But what their questions revealed was that touch and sound and taste, especially, were not sensory dimensions of the garden that were either usually verbalized or explicit. To the majority of gardeners touch, sound and taste, unlike sight and smell, remain parts of the sensory unconscious of gardening: there all the time but rarely acknowledged, thought about or discussed.

This apparent hierarchy of the importance of the different sensorial dimensions of gardening relates in an interesting way to the distance and relative degrees of intimacy of the garden in relation to the human body. The senses that do not require direct physical bodily contact (sight, sound and smell) are given greater verbal significance and acknowledgement than those that do (touch and taste).

While these sensory preferences did not significantly vary in relation to standard social variables such as income, occupation, nationality or age, or even experience or interest in gardening, there were some interesting gender differences. Although the visual experience of the garden was most important to both males and females (see Table 3) significantly more female gardeners than male gardeners

**Table 3.** The Significance of Different Sensory Dimensions of the Garden According to English Male (M) and Female (F) Gardeners

| Sensory dimension | Very important M% | Very important F% | Important M% | Important F% | Not important M% | Not important F% |
|---|---|---|---|---|---|---|
| Vision/appearance | 73 | 77 | 27 | 23 | 0 | 0 |
| Smell/scent | 35 | 46 | 54 | 49 | 11 | 5 |
| Touch/texture | 19 | 31 | 62 | 36 | 19 | 33 |
| Sound | 35 | 36 | 58 | 44 | 7 | 20 |
| Taste | 23 | 26 | 27 | 23 | 50 | 51 |

Number of informants = 65 of which males = 26 and females = 39

thought smell and touch to be very important to them and they were sometimes sensitized in relation to these experiential dimensions in a quite different way (see discussion below). Ten Swedish gardeners (16 percent) ranked all the senses (with the exception of taste in four cases) of equal importance. All but two of these were female and all had a high interest in gardening; it was their main or only hobby, most being members of gardening clubs. Eleven English gardeners (17 percent) similarly ranked all the senses (again with the exception of taste in three cases) as being of equal importance and eight of these (73 percent) were female.

**Vision**

"Its what's pleasing to the eye, you know. It's like looking at a pretty girl." (Male, 80, suburban gardener, Surrey, England.)

"Appearance [is the most important thing]. I do like having it laid out nicely." (Female, 40, South London allotment gardener.)

"In terms of my feeling for painting and what makes a good composition in painting, that is aesthetically satisfying, that has been used a great deal out there. I make sure, for example, that there are strong verticals. I love those plants that have a horizontal habit that look as if they are in layers and so on. [Both] give it a kind of grid structure … which is nice." (Male, 65, urban gardener, east London.)

"I always want to sit somewhere where I can be in a place where I like what I'm looking at. And where I get enormous visual pleasure out of what I look at." (Female, 59, urban gardener, north London.)

"I think it is very important to have an eye for design and it always rather annoys me when people have got a garden and they haven't bothered to design anything in it. It's all just hopelessly meandering. I don't mind it if it meanders purposefully." (Female, 74, urban gardener, west London.)

"I think its the visual, the look of it. I think probably the structure and the layout as well as color. I have really got big ideas that it is going to be full of flowers – it never is!" (Female, 54, urban gardener, Exeter, England.)

"You can paint with plants just like artists use pigment." (Female, 56, urban gardener, Dorset, England.)

"I think scent comes very fast after sight, but sight is first." It's the aspect that hits you, draws your attention to it, and then you want to go further." (Male, 73, gardener in modern housing estate, Dorset, England.)

"That's it [the garden] should be easily maintained and nice – nice to look at." (Female 46, suburban gardener, Halmstad, Sweden.)

"It takes two hours to go round [the garden]. Yes, it takes time! I'm very particular when I look at the plants. I take the flowers between the fingers of one hand and examine them. A leaf or flower isolated from their surroundings. That way you can really see them." (Male, 76, summerhouse gardener, Södermanland, Sweden.)

We have seen that for gardeners vision or sight dominates the overall perception of the garden, when forced to express this in words. This overriding significance of the visual aspect to the garden was explained by a few gardeners in a rather pragmatic manner. They pointed out that the visual appearance and color of the garden was of primary significance to them because you could see the garden from inside the house, and at all times and seasons. The other sensory aspects of the garden were not enduring or constant (scents and sounds come and go) and unlike vision they usually depended on you being physically out in the garden and among the plants. The appearance and color of the garden were said to be relaxing and pleasing to the eye whether you were in it or saw the garden from the house. For most, however, vision just *was* the dominant sense and did not require any further explication. For some vision was partly about garden design, i.e., form and structure, for others because the garden should look both pretty and be neat, tidy and well ordered. However, for most, vision was very strongly linked to an awareness of color and color combinations, hence the frequent references to painting, and the individual colors of flowers in particular.

### Color

"To begin with I realized that I didn't know very much about color, and I read so many distinguished gardeners, starting with Gertrude Jekyll, I suppose, who color-themed their gardens and nothing was out of place, nothing clashed, nothing did anything. And I thought, 'Oh God! I never think in these terms ...' And then I thought 'I don't care a stuff about color as far as this garden is concerned. I feel that those brilliant colors are the colors of the Mediterranean.' So I wanted strong reds and deep purples and yellows and it really didn't matter. And so I crammed them all in." (Male, 65, urban gardener, east London.)

"I'm more interested in the plant growth than the flowers – they're like the crown or the icing on the cake, but what's important to me is the plant itself. I look at the stem and the leaves." (Male, 75, suburban gardener, south Stockholm.)

"[In Regent's Park] there is a delphinium border, but it's got things before its delphinium stage. It's got lots of lilies and agapanthus and it's mostly blue and white with a bit of gray and yellow. It is sensitive. Next door to it, round the corner, is a begonia garden. It is absolutely embedded – red, orange, purple. It is absolutely hideous. It's got a little kind of Peter Pan in the middle. It is dire!" (Female, 59, urban gardener, north London.)

"Males tend to have stronger colors, clearer colors and more colors: strong reds, dark oranges and so on; women lighter, more variegated and muted colors.' (Male, 55, semi-rural summerhouse gardener, south Stockholm.)

"I'm not one of these people who must have a blue or white garden or a red and white garden or a corner in a particular color ... But no! I've found it has never offended anyone the way I have planted."
Chris: "So it's just a splash of color?"
"Yes, that's what I particularly like." (Male, 73, suburban gardener, Dorset, England.)

"We went to see a garden the other day by some famous fellow – Great Dixter [Christopher Lloyd's garden]. He's got this idea of putting strong colors together. It was quite fun, I suppose, but, you know, that's the sort of thing I think he does to shock – shocking colors. Well, I wouldn't like that." (Female, 68, urban gardener, west London.)

"If it's got color it's there, I think. I don't think I have any color bias really. I've just got a book on it [color in the garden] which I don't look at! I just see a plant and if it's a good color I buy it. I know it looks like I've color coordinated my petunias but I just bought the ones they had. So, no, all colors are welcome!" (Female, 46, urban gardener, Exeter, England.)

"I decided to restrict the color palette because I don't like clashing colors. I haven't got any yellow, or orange, not much red. It's all pinks, purple, bluey. I think that's more restful. I can't bear orange marigolds, red cannas. All those things I simply loathe." (Female, 74, urban gardener, west London.)

"It's not a busy garden. You can sit up the top there. It's a calm garden really. You've got pastel colours and it's not vibrant oranges and gnomes and petunias and so on. If you go in some gardens like the Park's Department you have got these different colors. You feel differently. Here, you can sit here and enjoy it. It's a calming garden, restful." (Male, 64, suburban gardener, Dorset, England.)

"In general my guiding principle is basically that it's either red foliage or red flowers, and by red I mean anything from the palest pink right through the reds to the darkest hues … One of the oriental things called Yin Yang is the theory of opposites. This is all part of the philosophy of opposites. So red being opposite green on the color circle, I'm only looking at color [in this way] … In the early spring/summer in particular you will see lots of red hydrangeas or azaleas and so forth. It's quite strong and that color comes out in Japan." (Male, 73, suburban gardener, Dorset, England.)

"Nothing too bright. No. I don't go in for bedding plants … Some gardens you pass by in the car and you almost need sunglasses to look at them because they're so florescent. You can see them from about three miles away!" (Female, 46, rural gardener, Wiltshire, England.)

"Have you seen this thing? [a bright red dahlia]. I think it is extraordinarily vulgar!"
Chris: "What is vulgar about it?"
"It's the size and the color. It's so vulgar it's really rather gorgeous isn't it? Well, yes. Maybe its just embarrassing. I don't know, but honestly *look* at that thing. I hadn't seen it until today. That must be a new one this year. I like those dark red things that are mixed with

pink [other dahlias] and it's a bit more subtle. But that! For God's sake! My husband will love that! He will really love it!" (Female, 59, rural gardener, Wiltshire, England.)

"I have got a blazing hot-colored vegetable garden because I think you need a bit of rock-and-roll with your pastoral music. Now and again you need to go and rock. You need a bit of shock and I love it. But I don't have bright bedding plants. It's exhausting. You don't want to look at it all of the time. I think I prefer the quiet music around." (Female, 56, rural gardener, Dorset, England.)

Color in the garden was considered by many to be the primary and most significant aspect of the visual appearance of the garden, so much so that garden design, form and structure tended to be thought of mostly in terms of color alone. It was very important to many gardeners to "keep the color" going throughout the year although most admitted it always tended to go "downhill" after August and that May and June were the best and brightest months. Color was spontaneously linked to a matter of "good taste" or "bad taste" in the garden by many. Color was of particular concern to female gardeners, while most male gardeners tended to be much less interested in it, remaining in many cases indifferent to supposed color "clashes." Differences in color preferences between gardeners are both heavily gendered and related to socioeconomic class, more so than most other aspects of gardening. These differences are structured according to a common set of dominant oppositions in which "good taste" refers, in the following list, to the right-hand column.

| bright | : | muted |
| bold | : | subtle |
| clashing | : | harmonious |
| random | : | themed |
| violent | : | restful |
| VULGAR | : | REFINED |

Brightly colored bedding plants and certain others, such as dahlias and gladioli with big flowers and bold colors, were banished from many gardens. They were often regarded by female gardeners of higher socioeconomic background in particular, as "common" and "vulgar" and "garish." However, such color sensibilities were quite often not recognized or shared by their male partners whose "vulgar" taste, arising either from ignorance or indifference, had to be excused. Women of lower socioeconomic class had, like most males, a much less judgmental and less opinionated view about color either saying, in response to the question: "Is color important to you in your garden?" such things as "Oh yes! It's nice with a bit of color," or "If you've got color it brightens the day." It clearly didn't matter what kind of color this was or the kind of plant that happened to be flowering or which plant it was next to. Most males felt that women were much more interested in flowers in general, and colors in particular than they were themselves. While they appreciated flowers they claimed that they were much more interested in the plant itself throughout the year, the different forms of the leaves and shades of green. Subtle shades of color in the garden were claimed to be both restful and peaceful, usually by female gardeners, and to have a therapeutic and calming effect, as opposed to a *riot* of color that was disturbing and upsetting.

Ideas about color, and its appropriateness or not, were heavily influenced by knowledge of gardening and belonging, or not, to a social network of other gardeners, and related to age: the older the gardener, the more conservative their views tended to be. Thus color was only a difficult problem to be confronted and intellectually dealt with, (or reconciled in some way with what they had actually planted in their gardens) by those who had read a lot about gardening in books and magazines and/or personally knew many other keen gardeners through membership of gardening societies. Here opinions were often very heavily influenced by concepts of different styles of garden, or the history of gardening, e.g. the Victorian love of brightly colored bedding plants in municipal parks and gardens, or that the creation of a Mediterranean-style garden in England required bright (brash to some) colors and whether such colors and types of gardens in England might be deemed appropriate or not. A minority of gardeners thought that different colors were best at different seasons of the years, yellow for example being more appropriate in the spring than in the stronger light of summer.

For many, almost always those with either little knowledge of or interest in gardens, or both, concepts of "vulgarity" in relation either to different kinds of plants or colors were completely absent. They liked parks and private gardens to be full of flowers, of whatever kind, and "showy." Thus a conscious and deliberate concern with color is primarily a self-invented "problem" of the bourgeoisie, which through interest and reading, is also acquired and reproduced as a dominant ethos, or set of values and aspirations, by those of lower socioeconomic status.

### Smell

"Scent: it smells of home." (Female 44, rural gardener, Södermanland, Sweden.)

"I like my garden to smell nice, smell of … garden … I cook. Smell is important in cooking, a nice smell, in my garden, like after the rain comes, I like to smell the plants from my garden, smell even in the summer when it's hot and dusty." (Male, 52, allotment gardener, south London.)

"The idea of the scented garden is the ultimate." (Female, 54, rural gardener, Dorset, England)

"For girls scent is often very important. For men, well, they're not so interested." (Male 55, semi-rural gardener, south Stockholm.)

"I have lilies. They let out such a wonderful scent. Beguiling. It leaks out." (Female, 84, suburban gardener, Lund, Sweden.)

"I've got some azaleas which come from South America that have a wonderful perfume and even if you were blind you'd know they were there. You don't find that with so many roses now. I think it's a pity really." (Male, 80, suburban gardener, Surrey.)

"[Scent is] very important. Did you know that the smell of certain things can make you healthy: that sage there, the smell of the stuff, it can make you healthy." (Female, 69, allotment gardener, South London.)

"A good scent will stop me in my tracks. I'll want to know where it is coming from… [The freshly dug] soil, it smells wonderful and it looks so good. If it is really good soil you know when you turn it over. Because of the smell and the texture and the way it falls. One of the best smells in the garden is when you have had a long, hot, dry period and it rains. All the plants smell and the soil smells and the tarmac and the paving slabs. It's wonderful! There's nothing like wet tarmac after a dry period!" (Female, 56, urban gardener, Dorset, England.)

"Most people when they see a beautiful flower, you will see them go forward and smell it and sometimes you'll see the look of disappointment when nothing is forthcoming." (Male, 73, suburban gardener in modern housing estate, Dorset, England.)

"I'm just appalled at how people just don't know how to release the fragrance of the plant. You have to actually show them that you rub the leaf and smell it because people bend down to sniff the leaf … And it's such a revelation to them." (Female, 46, rural gardener, Wiltshire, England)

"I think the sense of smell is very important because it is so incredibly evocative. Your whole life, you can smell where you are … the sort of smell I love is the sort of Italian smell, the spicy scent of pine trees and things like that." (Female, 72, rural gardener, Dorset, England.)

When talking about scent gardeners mentioned a wide variety of different experiences: the smell of the earth itself, the smoke of bonfires, the smell of rain after a dry spell, of newly mown grass, compost and, of course, the sweet scents of particularly loved plants such as honeysuckle, jasmine, roses, herbs, night-scented stock and tobacco plants. Some gardeners complained that hybrid roses were now being cultivated primarily for their form and color and that all the scent, characteristic of old-fashioned, "inferior" and disease-prone roses had been bred out of the new fancy varieties (cf. Classen 1993). While smell was important to some English allotment owners, who were primarily growing vegetables, they generally felt they had less of it than other gardeners, because of the lack of flowers. However, smell could be a general rather than specific sensation: gardens might have their own smell, just as houses or landscapes or cars had theirs.

Scent was particularly important to many gardeners both because it let them know that they were in the garden and through this experience they felt that they became more an intimate part of it. Smell or scent differentiated between the inside and the outside of the house. It signaled and highlighted the *individual* character of different plants, which became more alive with their own distinctive scents and textures as real living things. While from the house vision revealed the garden as being like a painting – a visual representation, seen from a particular point of view, the bedroom window, or the living room door – being in it and smelling the plants emphasized the garden as something very different, a living and changing thing.

**Touch**

"I'd never thought of touch and texture. I don't think I go round the garden feeling things. But there are mossy stones and smooth stones, but I hadn't thought whether they were important or not." (Female, 58, rural gardener, Devon, England.)

"I love handling soil and leaves and stones. The touch of everything and the fragrances and the whole thing is sublime." (Female, 56, rural gardener, Dorset, England.)

"Touch and texture. I love working with the soil, so a lot of it's that." (Female, 40, allotment gardener, South London.)

"Texture and touch is a very sensual thing. The texture you want to touch ... You know: touching things that you really admire, that you are curious about." (Female, 56, urban gardener, Dorset, England.)

"I love to touch the plants because then you understand them more." (Female, 55, rural gardener, Devon, England.)

"Its hard to get a feeling of touch – a pleasurable feeling of touch – from flowers ... Just to touch a flower like this wouldn't do much for me." (Male, 73, suburban gardener, Dorset, England.)

"I wear gloves when I'm doing mucky wet stuff, otherwise I don't." (Female, 62, rural gardener, Devon, England.)

"Gloves? No, they're a hindrance to me. I had some nail extensions for my wedding but you see they're all coming off, because I can't." (Female, 66, rural gardener, Devon, England.)

"When I was in America I got attacked by poison ivy. Now I've got an allergy to any kind of ivy, so if I happen to brush up against any in the garden I've got a rash that lasts three weeks. I've just got over one now. But no! Look, I'm a gardener. You can't pick up most weeds with gloves." (Male, 66, rural gardener, Dorset, England.)

"I have started to wear rubber gloves. But my nails are an absolute disgrace and I've just started to try and look after them a bit more … But I'm sure they'll go to pot when I get my hands in the soil and I can't get on with gloves when I really get stuck in. I can't be bothered." (Female, 46, rural gardener, Wiltshire, England.)

"I find it heartbreaking because I dress myself up to the nines and suddenly I look at my hands and I think "Oh no! I've been gardening. If I start with gloves I soon take them off and spend the rest of the time looking for them." (Female, 70, urban gardener, Dorset, England.)

"I dig the compost with my hands. I always work without gloves because I want to feel the soil. It's important!" (Female, 52, suburban gardener, Halmstad, Sweden.)

Touch bears a much more intimate relationship to the body than sight or sound or smell. Gardening is primarily working with the hands, and some gardeners even liked to dig freshly turned soil with their hands when planting out rather than using tools, or would scoop out a drill for seeds with their fingers. Gardeners have dirty and frequently scarred hands. When I asked whether they thought people could have "green fingers" a standard joke was "I don't know about that. Mine are usually black!" Touching plants was an important aspect of gardening to most gardeners. Although most did not rate this sensation highly in relation to the other senses, being able to touch and feel the plants was, in fact, incredibly important to them. Over and over, people commented that they "liked to touch the plants." It was to the leaves and bark, and the soil, rather than the flowers, that they were primarily referring as flowers tend to be thought of, almost exclusively, in terms of color and form.

All but a few gardeners of both sexes possessed one or more pairs of gardening gloves. One female gardener wore them all the time because she did not like the feel of soil on her hands. She was very much the exception. Most gardeners rarely wore gloves, or forgot they had any, or were continually losing them in the garden. They liked to feel the soil and the plants and most claimed it was impossible to carry out tasks such as weeding with gloves on. Some gardeners even preferred to dig holes when planting out plants in pots with their hands rather than using a trowel and they liked to feel the soil as they put it around the plants. One male Swedish gardener even dug a large hole and planted a quite substantial tree in this fashion; others dug and mixed compost with their bare hands. So gloves remained neglected and unused except for certain highly specific tasks such as removing stinging nettles, brambles or pruning roses, and even then they were frequently forgotten. Wearing gloves made gardeners feel clumsy and out of proper physical contact with the plants and the soil.

Feeling the damp soil, the texture of the leaves, the bark of trees and shrubs was an essential part of the intimate experience of gardening, but this sensation was often very difficult to express in words. Seeing and smelling things, as often as not, led to a desire to touch them, to physically experience them through the hands, cupping the rosebud while smelling it, or bruising the leaves of herbs and other aromatic plants in order to coax the scent out of them onto the fingers. Another aspect of touch that was mentioned was through the feet, the delicious sensation of walking on the grass with bare feet, especially when dew-laden on a summer's morning. Most gardeners had favorite tools, and what they particularly liked about them was the way they felt in their hands as extensions of their bodies. Interestingly, weeding was a favorite task for a substantial number of Swedish and English female gardeners, but was rarely liked by males. One of the reasons given for the joy of weeding was that it provided intimate contact with the plants: "You come down at the level of the ground, kneel down and weed. You come down to the same level as the plants and can feel the scent and find seedlings and look after them" (female, 68, suburban gardener, Eskilstuna, Sweden).

## Sound

"Not really. I don't go for bamboos and swishing grasses." (Female, 27, allotment gardener, south London.)

"Sound, the peace and quiet … so it's not really sound, its like silence rather." (Female 39, allotment gardener, south London.)

"I love the sound of bamboo. And the sound of the wind in the trees. You know, they affect the senses far more than just color I think … If you shut your eyes the sound is still there, so it's much more physical than merely looking at something." (Female 56, urban gardener, Dorset, England.)

"I think [I most enjoy the] sound really. It's the peace of the garden that one appreciates. Although what I really appreciate like mad is bird life. And I think that is absolutely everything. Particularly in the early spring or even in the mid spring I often go out there just to hear the dawn chorus. That's gorgeous." (Male, 73, suburban gardener, Dorset, England)

"Sound is very important. You will have calm and harmony in your garden." (Female, 47, Bjärred, suburban gardener, Sweden.)

"I don't understand those who go out with a strimmer or motor lawn mower. It is so disturbing. It should be a nice sound. Bird song. I like to smell the flowers, not the smell of petrol." (Female 45, suburban gardener, Halmstad, Sweden.)

"You shouldn't have music in the garden. It should be quiet. Only nature should speak." (Female 84, suburban gardener, Lund, Sweden)

Sound was almost always considered in two contrasting ways, either as unpleasant and unwanted, or as delightful and needed. To some sound was primarily annoying, intrusive and unwanted: road noise, low-flying jets, noisy neighbors. Complaints about the noise made by neighbors and their garden machinery were common among Swedish gardeners but, curiously, rarely mentioned by English gardeners. Such unwanted noises were generally considered disturbing and the garden as a "natural" thing should necessarily soothe the soul. A garden should ideally exclude such unwanted and unnatural noise. It should be calm and quiet enough to enable pleasant "natural" sounds to be encountered. These might be expected to be different every time one went into it depending on the breeze, or the wind, and its direction, the time of year, the different species of birds and insects that might be attracted to dwell within it. Sound, in particular, signified life in the garden, the garden as a living thing rather than as an inanimate object. To some, especially rural gardeners, the presence of sound was usually the result of some kind of animation: running water, the movement of the wind, of birds, the barking of a dog, or the cries of playing children.

The one desirable feature most frequently mentioned by both English and Swedish gardeners that might turn their existing garden into a dream garden was the presence of water – a large pond or, preferably, running water, a small stream with a waterfall. Importantly it was the relaxing sound of water as much as its visual appearance that was the most significant factor.

## Taste
"That is the most important thing ... mainly for the taste." (Male, 73, allotment gardener, south London.)

"Taste is very important ... [fresh from the allotment] the taste is much better." (Female, 60, allotment gardener, south London.)

"I'm more interested in growing it than in eating it." (Female, 40, allotment gardener, south London.)

The significance accorded to taste in the garden was usually directly related to more practical interests in the garden. A majority of English and Swedish gardeners were not growing any fruit or vegetables at all, or only had symbolic, token plots or one or two fruit trees, and, as a result, taste was insignificant to them. As might be expected taste was far more important to allotment gardeners growing significant quantities of fruit and vegetables than someone with a lawn and flower beds. If people did grow fruit and vegetables they all stated that it was primarily for the freshness and the taste. Among south London allotment gardeners taste was ranked as very important by three out of the six gardeners interviewed with only one attributing to it no significance at all. Similarly, taste was of greater importance for other allotment owners outside London, in Sweden and for English rural gardeners (29 percent of whom ranked taste as very important), who were far more likely to be growing significant quantities of fruit and vegetables than urban or suburban gardeners. So clearly there is a pragmatic interest here in the manner in which the various senses are thought to be important.

But the taste of your own fruit and vegetables was often linked to a concern to grow organic vegetables without using pesticides or artificial fertilizers. Equally important was labor, the love, care and attention devoted to cultivation. Simply because they had grown them the crops would be eaten whatever their size and appearance. A sprout the size of a pea would be eaten because they had grown it, or a split parsnip root only a few centimeters long. An obsession with the shape and size (i.e. the visual aspect) of fruit and vegetables is peculiarly shared both by supermarkets and a small minority of gardeners involved in competitive exhibiting at garden shows.

## Synesthetic Experience

It was in particular the intimacy of scent, touch and sound that some gardeners emphasized as being very important to them: value was placed on wandering in the garden and being surprised, encountering the unexpected and experiencing difference. The more intimate of the senses had evocative powers in relation to memory. They could transport gardeners to different places and times and transcend the present state of being in a particular garden and in a particular place. Most maintained that smell, scent and sound gave moments of "extra pleasure" when going round the garden, which must primarily please and satisfy the eye first because this, unlike the other senses, gave both instant and long-lasting satisfaction. More effort was generally required in relation to the other senses. However, these sensory dimensions might heighten the intimacy and depth of feeling in a garden in a manner that vision could not.

Gardeners, like the rest of us, lack a sophisticated vocabulary to talk about sounds or scents or touch or taste compared with the way in which we can readily talk about visual aspects of the garden, or it can be argued, such sensations are so all-embracing and personally intimate they become part of our unconscious. The prime importance that gardeners explicitly attribute to sight is not very surprising. Many scholars have commented that we live in a contemporary culture of vision. Some historians and anthropologists have argued that in different cultures, in the past or in other parts of the world, other bodily senses such as sound or smell have been more important than sight (e.g. Ong 1982; Stoller 1989; Classen 1993; Howes 1991). In relation to gardening, it has been the case that the scents of certain flowers, such as the rose, were far more significant in the past (Classen 1993). All the recent emphasis has been on cultivating for color and resistance to diseases (the latter leading to a diminishment of scent). It is interesting to note that such is the significance of the visual in contemporary Western culture that of all the senses it stands alone as a sensory signifier of "good" or "bad" taste in the garden for some. Nobody ever mentioned vulgarity in relation to touch, smell, sound or taste.

Garden form and design, color and shape, are all discussed, of course, at great length in popular books on gardening and gardens as are sweet-scented and aromatic plants such as herbs and the taste of fresh fruit and vegetables. By comparison there are very few discussions of either touch or sound in the garden. Indeed there are only a handful of popular gardening books that explicitly draw attention to the differing sensory dimensions of the garden in an explicit manner (e.g. Cox 1993; Don 1997; Brunton and Fournier 1999). In this respect the gardening literature displays a similar sensory lacuna to that expressed by the gardeners I talked to in relation to taste and touch, scent and sound, while over and over again the dominant emphasis is on the visual aspect of the garden. The bodily senses that seem to be most important to gardeners are almost in inverse relationship to their intimacy.

A small minority of gardeners did, however, explicitly mention the manner in which certain of the senses overlapped and mingled when you are out in the garden. The manifold intimate sensory dimensions of the garden were innumerable and inseparable, and furthermore many were not deliberately designed by the gardener, they just occurred of their own accord:

"I think that is one of the magic things about gardening. You see the plants and can listen to the birds. There is the visual and the aural." (Male, 66 rural gardener, Dorset, England.)

"Wafts of smell stop one in one's tracks. There is a sense of sweetness and also of other things going on, changes in color are part of things moving with the seasons." (Female, 60, rural gardener, Devon, England).

"To have some scented flowers is important. There is also the smell of rain, of rotting compost, of freshly cut grass. Touch: spiky, hairy, smoothness, nettles, the dew on the grass. Sound: the crunch of gravel, of the spade when digging, bird song, horrible sounds: the traffic." (Male, 46, rural gardener, Dorset, England.)

"I can't divide up all those different senses. They're all important. In the beginning it wasn't so. It was only the visual that was important – color and form in relationship to each other. Just as at the beginning you only look at the flowers and then you realize there are other aspects to the plant all year round. It's not just interesting for a week. For me all the senses are important, although taste isn't so important. I don't bother with that. For me colors, form and structure, the visual that's primary, and to feel. Scent is secondary, but I will rather have plants with scent if they are available. I have analyzed all this with myself and most people don't consciously think of all the senses. I think they are all important but you don't normally think of these things. If I should choose a rose for my garden it should be scented." (Female, 45, suburban gardener, south Stockholm.)

"Smell, scent, lets me know I'm in a garden and gives the plants character. It's quite an intimate thing, like texture. Feeling/smelling the plants is important because they become more alive to me. Their is an element of ownership, oddly, and it creates a boundary between inside (where I live mostly) and outside – things that lie outside have their own scent and texture and I appreciate the difference' (Female, 46, urban gardener, Exeter, England.)

Gardening is practical, work carried out with the hands and through the body – embodied activity: doing rather than saying and most gardeners prefer to work rather than talk about what they are doing. In fact not having to talk about what they were doing or feeling was one of the primary attractions of gardening. It provided an escape from verbal discourse. It is the intimacy of bodily contact through all the senses, rarely put into words, or even thought about, that can be readily observed when you study the manner in which gardeners actually garden. All, or most of, the senses are in fact very significant to the vast majority of gardeners all of the time, but this almost always goes relatively unacknowledged in their words. However, it can be observed in their practice: how they actually garden and care for the plants, and the manner in which they walk about their gardens and remark about particular things in them. Conversations about flower colors typically rapidly turn to note the presence of a song bird, or the presence of a sticky patch of soil here, or the sweet taste of a particular variety of raspberries there, or the heady scent of a lily.

For most gardeners the taste of fruit and vegetables is intimately connected with their smell and form. They will ordinarily bruise the leaves of aromatic plants to release their smell, or cup a rose in the palm of their hands to feel the scent of the petals. A garden without bird song or the buzzing sounds of insects would seem instantly peculiar to most. Shapes are frequently noted that are entirely created by colors and variations in light and shade. Vegetables taste nice partly because they are grown in neat and tidy rows, a well-tilled soil feels and smells and sounds and looks exhilarating. Gardeners sense the garden with their entire bodies, most of the time, and these sensory experiences always mingle and overlap. The multidimensional and synthesthetic sensory experiences of the garden thus become part and parcel of the entire process of gardening rather than experiences that are analytically abstracted and separated from each other.

## Conclusions

The sensory feeling for the garden is deeper and much more profound than most gardeners can, will (for fear of sounding silly), or do acknowledge. Such synesthetic experience was frequently implicitly expressed by the use of the term "harmony": "Relax. That's why I have a garden. To feel the harmony in my garden" (male, 45. Suburban gardener, Halmstad, Sweden). The garden to him, and many others, should ideally be a harmonious multisensorial mixture of plants and other features that soothe the soul, something that relieves anxiety and provides a calming and therapeutic experience as opposed to the stresses of working life.

The everyday phenomenological significance of the garden, in this respect, is that its experience is primordial and non-reflectively, or discursively, embodied, blowing apart any modernist categorizations of the senses into supposedly separate and discrete spheres of human experience and perception. Thus the ontological significance of gardening in contemporary modernity is that it reconnects us with that which has become artificially fragmented in both our intellectual and increasingly urbanized culture. Our primordial relationship with the garden is through our sensing and sensed carnal bodies, a world of embodied perception in which we are not separate from the garden around us. Gardening thus provides a primary medium for people to escape from an interior sensory world increasingly defined by the limits of the plate-glass window. It is a place in which millions of people actively labor in order to experience the delight of the full human intimacy of their sensuous carnal being. The relationship between gardener and garden is thus truly akin to that between lovers.

## References

Buchli, V. (ed.). 2002. *The Material Culture Reader*. Oxford: Berg.

Bull, M. and Back, L. (eds). 2003. *The Auditory Culture Reader*. Oxford: Berg.

Brunton, L. and Fournier, E. 1999. *Sanctuary: Gardening for the Soul*. New York: Michael Friedman

Classen, C. 1993. "The Odour of the Rose. Floral Symbolism and the Olfactory Decline of the West." In C. Classen *Worlds of Sense: Exploring the Senses in History and Across Cultures*. London: Routledge.

——. 1993. *Worlds of Sense: Exploring the Senses in History and Across Cultures*. London: Routledge.

—— (ed.) 2005. *The Book of Touch*. Oxford: Berg.

Cox, J. 1993. *Creating a Graden for the Senses*, New York: Abbeville Press

Don, M. 1997. *The Sensuous Garden*. London: Conran Octopus.

Howes, D (ed.). 1991. *The Varieties of Sensory Experience*. Toronto: University of Toronto Press.

—— (ed.). 2005. *Empire of the Senses*. Oxford: Berg.

Howes, D. 2006. "Scent, Sound and Synaesthesia: Intersensoriality and Material Culture Theory." In C. Tilley, W. Keane, S. Kuechler, M. Rowlands and P. Spyer (eds.), *Handbook of Material Culture*. London: Sage.

Marcus, G. 1995. "Ethnography in/of the World System: The Emergence of Multi-sited Ethnography." *Annual Review of Anthropology* 24: 95–117.

Ong, W. 1982. *Orality and Literacy: The Technologizing of the World*. London: Methuen.

Stoller, P. 1989. *The Taste of Ethnographic Things: The Senses in Anthropology*. Philadelphia: University of Pennsylvania Press.

Tilley, C. 2001. "Ethnography and Material Culture." In P. Atkinson, A. Colley, S. Delamont, J. Lofland and L. Lofland (eds), *Handbook of Ethnography*. London: Sage.

——. 2004. *The Materiality of Stone: Explorations in Landscape Phenomenology*. Oxford: Berg.

Tilley, C. Keane, W., Kuchler, S., Rowlands, M and Spyer, P. (eds). 2006. *Handbook of Material Culture*. London: Sage.

# Learning How to Listen
## Kroncong Music in a Javanese Neighborhood

### Steve Ferzacca

Steve Ferzacca received his Ph.D. from the University of Wisconsin-Madison (1996) in Anthropology and Southeast Asian Studies. He continues ethnographic fieldwork in the Indonesian city of Yogyakarta on topics that include urban medicine, psychological anthropology and expressive culture. He is currently working on a new book that examines the cultural history of Javanese emotivity. steven.ferzacca@uleth.ca.

ABSTRACT   In this article I consider several weeks of music rehearsals that took place in an urban neighborhood in the Indonesian city of Yogyakarta. The music "rehearsed" by a group of men is kroncong; an urban folk music incorporating a string band, flute, vocals and sometimes a keyboard that in Indonesia dates to the arrival of the Portuguese and the establishment of urban enclaves of traders and slaves in the sixteenth century along the north coast of Java. The melancholy and other historically anchored sensorial sentiments evoked by the totality of sound and image that comprises the songs, as well as the activities and associations that go into making kroncong music, are referred to as kroncong *sensibilia*. The discussion of sensibilia follows an analytical path that begins with the poetics of the musical genre and moves on to an examination of the politics of kroncong sensibilia in a particular context of social relations. For the Javanese men of the neighborhood, the making of kroncong music was at one level a nostalgic response to their urban lives. However, perhaps more importantly, making kroncong music was a tactical and strategic act of sound and sentiment, a particularly masculine one, seeking "recognition" within an "aesthetic community" and built world of social relations increasingly organized around and by, if not centered on, women.

### Learning How to Listen

To live in an urban Javanese neighborhood, known as *kampung*, is to open up oneself to an empire of sounds and a syntagm of phonic signs. The kampung as a built world of sound, its acoustical features, timbres and pitch resounding the patterns and rhythms of everyday social life, is illustrative of how sound structure reflects social structure (Feld 1982: 14–15), and, in this case, how complexes of sound (syntagm) gain illocutionary force within an aural grammar of social relations (empire). In Rumah Putri (a pseudonym), the urban kampung in Yogyakarta, Indonesia where I have conducted fieldwork since 1992, these soundings of daily life only began to make sense to me after some time had passed, and after my attunements to this soundscape depreciated under the spell of familiarity. I learned to tune out the call to prayer from the local *mesjid* (mosque) early in the pre-dawn morning, followed by the rustlings of pots and the steam of boiling rice, the crowing of cocks, splashes of bathwater, the rhythmic clip-clop of flip-flops, the musical advertisements of roving prepared-food vendors, flourishes of children's voices fading off towards school, pulsating *dangdut* music adding rhythm to morning chores, cackling hens and chirping chicks scrounging for something to eat and the bustle of men and women off to work and the market.

I stopped listening to the aural cadence of fading mornings into afternoons, and the kampung quiets, underscored again with the call for prayer and sputtering motorbikes. Small children and women appear from inside their homes to talk and fancy the musical parade of food. A kind of lazy quietude until other sounds – the swish of bamboo brooms cleaning the public dust and clutter of the day, followed by the splashes of water – herald the arrival of late afternoon. Then, a jamboree of all-over social life breaks out as kampung residents congregate in the lanes and back streets out in front of or near their homes for *sore*, the late afternoon social time valued by kampung residents. Escaping from behind closed doors of those who own televisions the laugh tracks and dialogue of

Indonesian *cinetron* (sitcoms) spill out through the thin walls falling upon ears of envy. Night approaches, the call for prayer returns and the sounds of people are carried into their homes as they eat and take their evening bath. An occasional radio news program mixes in with the chatter of dinnertime. With nightfall the re-emergent laughter and talk fill the streets along with the sputter of motorbikes. Groups shuffle along on their way to prayer meetings. Polite greetings are exchanged by congregates and passers-by. As evening proceeds the pitch of sociality builds. Youths, young men and women, begin to gather together to gossip, romance, and play music. Middle-aged men smoke and dream, while their wives and small children relive their day. As nine o'clock approaches, women and children return to their homes. The murmurs of men are overwhelmed by the croons of youths singing Indonesian pop songs and fractured American hits at the top of their lungs. After midnight the murmurings of men, the lusty songs of romantic youth and the lizard songs of the gecko dovetail into the all-night radio broadcasts of shadow-puppet performances with bell percussions of gamelan music punctuated by the verbal gymnastics of puppeteers. Then it all begins again.

 I had learned to tune out these soundings of social life – until one evening when a new embellishment was added to my muted soundscape. Just before the sun set, I noticed that a group of men had arrived at a neighbor's house with musical instruments: guitars, a string bass, an electric keyboard, a viola, a flute and a microphone with an amplifier. On other nights to follow an occasional banjo and ukulele joined the ensemble. The musicians were newcomers, outsiders to kampung. Several of my neighbors walked past me towards the house and explained that there were going to be *latihan* (rehearsals) of kroncong music at Pak Wayang's house. Soon after, the strums of guitar, the cry of a violin, the plucking of acoustic bass and the stylized vocals of *kroncong* music loudly disturbed the round of sounds. The rehearsals lasted about a month and as suddenly as they had appeared they disappeared. From over the shoulders of my neighbors I detected no excitement or fuss about the appearance or disappearance of the kroncong rehearsals. This fleeting addition to the soundscape of kampung life was not marked in any way, or so I thought.

 In this essay I want to consider those weeks of kroncong rehearsals on the porch of Pak Wayang's home as the basis for a study in social relations.[1] In this Javanese kampung, the making of kroncong music was both an aesthetic and practical activity meant to be recognized as a part of neighborhood social relations at large. If the making of kroncong music can tell us something of the social lives of men and women in this kampung, I suggest that the making kroncong music *is* the making of social lives.[2]

 As many have shown us, expressive forms of culture, songs, poetry, dance, oral and literary works, often provide the opportunity to "stretch parameters of everyday speech … to extraordinary

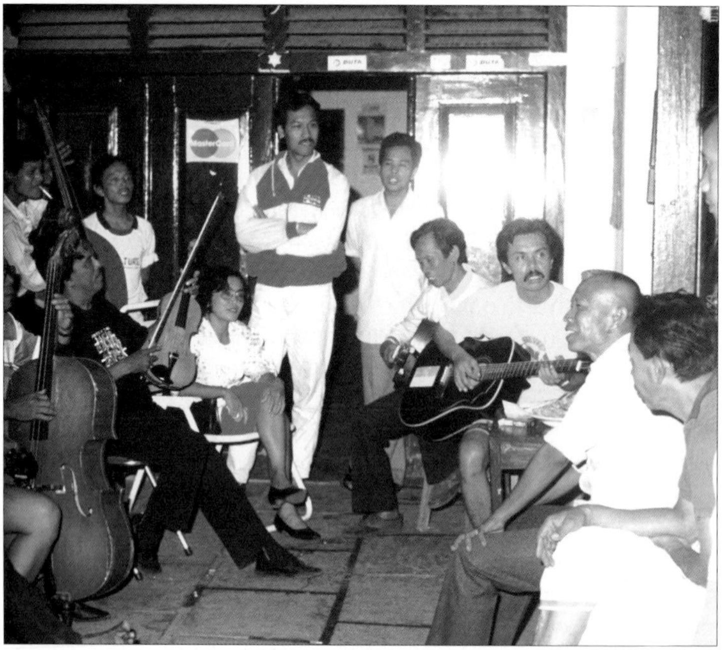

**Figure 1**
Kroncong rehearsal.
Photograph:
Steve Ferzacca

dimensions, enabling sentiments and values otherwise suppressed or ineffable to take momentary shape" (Roseman 1996: 233).[3] Making kroncong music represents just such a "stretch," and does so with soundful sentiments that for many Javanese are valued as worthy of remembering. I will refer to these sensorial sentimentalities deemed to be both memorable and worthwhile as *sensibilia*. For the men who gathered on the porch across the way making kroncong music was at one level a nostalgic response to their urban lives. However, on a perhaps more important, deeper level, making kroncong music was, as I see it, a tactical and strategic act of sound and sentiment, a particularly masculine one, seeking recognition (Keane 1997:9) within an "aesthetic community" (Goldstein 1995:312) and built world of social relations increasingly organized around and by, if not centered on women. On those cool evenings in Rumah Putri, making kroncong music was about making gender and class, and so the "musicking" of social life in this Javanese kampung.

### Kroncong Sensibilia

Kroncong sensibilia are the sensorial sentiments evoked by the totality of sound and image that comprise the songs, but also by the activities and associations that go into making kroncong music that are meant to "move" people as well.[4] Briefly, these kroncong sensibilia embody and express the emotionally charged irony of human love and longing for love lost and found, a cosmopolitan, urban history, various relationships to a particular modernity and other modern moments in the awakening of the Indonesian national imagination, a nostalgia for the past and the pastoral forged from historical and a local sense of syncretic authenticity and invention. These sensibilia, considered on their own, however, are insufficient towards an understanding of how making music is a study in social relations. The discussion of sensibilia here follows an analytical path that begins with the poetics of the musical genre and moves onto an examination of the politics of kroncong sensibilia in a particular context of social relations. So the path is from kroncong as cultural production to kroncong as social practice. With this framework in mind the kroncong sensibilia include the affective quality of its sound, its sense of places, the histories it embodies, the memories it arouses, the cultural biographies (Kopytoff 1986) it conveys, the social lives it has lived. As an instrument in the making of social relations, kroncong sensibilia become useful for the evocation of particular social identities that make sense in particular networks and contexts. Small (1998) considers such "musicking" (p.2) of social life, as ritual activity through which music makers and listeners enact social identities. The kroncong rehearsals I observed functioned similarly as aural modes of social interaction within the historically constituted particularities of kampung social life and society. In Rumah Putri, the puppet maker and the men who chose to join in the kroncong rehearsals were drawing upon other sensibilia related to this genre of music, specifically its association with a dangerous, virile sense of masculinity. In addition, these men also attempted to associate this musicking with an unrelated masculine sensibilia culturally and socially significant for a Javanese noble character historically anchored in Javanese gender relations forged in the context of court society. This novel configuration reveals that considerations of cultural productions not in use may be unable to predict their meaning and the experience of their meaning in locally constituted social activity.

## Sounds like Modernity

In 1850, on a visit to the south coast of Java, Sir Francis Drake encountered kroncong music and described it as "a very strange kind" of "country musick", with a "pleasant and delightful" sound (Kunst 1973: 5). Kroncong music is string-band music that features an ensemble of guitars, ukuleles, banjos, viola, string bass or 'cello, flute, and vocals, and perhaps a keyboard.[5] Kroncong in Indonesia dates to the arrival of the Portuguese and the establishment of urban enclaves of traders and slaves in the sixteenth century along the north coast of Java. Kroncong shares a heritage with the "urban folk music" of Portugal known as *fado*.[6] In Portugal fado music is considered a national music and emerged as a song-form during the Moorish occupation before the Crusades.[7] Vernon

(1998: 6) suggests that fado most likely took its name from a group known as the *Faditas* (fatalists) who sang and wrote fado songs. Both fado and kroncong are cultural products of global flows and "ethnoscapes." In Indonesia kroncong was first played by ethnic mix of urban dwellers that included "Indo-European populations" (Kunst 1973: 375), "Eurasians" (Kornhauser 1978:104), "Africans, Indians, and Malays" (Sumarsam 1992: 19) and other "mestico (mestizo) persons" (Tsuchiya 1989: 11) who inhabited the urban kampungs of these trading port cities. Kroncong's musical elements continue to sound these and later cultural encounters as well as subsequent periods of change in the developing Indonesian imagination.

Kroncong in Indonesia is usually considered a "syncretic," "acculturated," or "hybrid" art form of expressive culture in which "non-Western" (the two-scale systems of gamelan music and percussive instruments) and "Western elements" (string instruments and diatonic scale) converge to produce "a unified combination of stylistic sources in the one art product" (ibid.). Over time, in Java, kroncong has combined musical elements from other local musical genres, particularly gamelan (Lockhard 1998: 63). While some Indonesian kroncong artists claim its authenticity as a uniquely Indonesian musical genre, its growth in popularity during the period of national awakening and Independence was to a great degree due to its "international character" and dynamic inclusive capacity – a "collective Indonesian music" that sounded the collective Indonesian imagined community in-the-making (Sumarsam 1992: 119–120).

In the late nineteenth and early twentieth centuries kroncong music found its most devoted audience in the Eurasian populations and among the lower classes of urban kampung (Kornhauser 1978: 131), and became an "urban folk music of the proletariat" (Heins 1975: 21). Tsuchiya (1989:19) argues that it is precisely this "otherness" that later on was important for the association of kroncong with Indonesian nationalist projects. Becker (1975), Kornhauser (1978), and Sumarsam (1992) briefly outline the *rise* of kroncong as a "national" music, and for contemporary Indonesia Yampolsky (1989:10) lists kroncong among several other "national music genres."[8] Certainly kroncong music's prominent place in the sensibilia of Indonesian nationalism as the sound and sentiment of protest, revolution and independence is significant, particularly in light of the positioning of kroncong, during nation building, with other musical genres. In the heady days of the nationalist movement the role of musical and theatrical genres in nationalist rhetoric were debated as to their appropriateness as markers of *Indonesian* identity (Sumarsam 1992: 119). In its search for a country, kroncong music, without its ties to any one ethnic group or tradition, became an expression of the revolutionary spirit, and found a country within the spirit of Indonesian independence and the "unity in diversity" of the Indonesian nation-state. Kroncong, like Bahasa Indonesia the Malay language that was chosen to become the national language, represents a lingua franca of exchange that attempts to transcend difference rather than mark it through specific ethnic affiliations. In this way the sound of kroncong is an auditory sign of a new and emerging kind of "modern" society, representing a rupture with traditional relations of rank and circumstance and the appearance of a new age.

Kroncong's association with low-class, urban kampung dwellers, particularly low-class men, continues to charge kroncong sensibilia in spite of the loss of some of this tarnish, especially recently (Lockhard 1998:64). As Lockhard (1998), Becker (1975), Yampolsky (1991) and others note, kroncong musicians were mostly men whose attributes were less than savory. Often characterized as unsettled, wandering, sexual *buaya* (crocodiles) on the prowl, kroncong musicians involved themselves in the numerous sins that aroused a sense of danger, cunning, virility and spontaneity that many Javanese simultaneously find appealing but at the same time fearful. This "déclassé, disrespectable image" (Lockhard 1998: 64) of the kroncong musician becomes revised with its emerging association as the sound of modernity and Indonesian nationalism and its commercial successes propelled by its dominance in radio broadcasts, film scores, and later television.[9] As we will see in the Rumah Putri rehearsals this kroncong sensibilia is a recognizably transgressive, even parodic, feature in my estimation of this music making as a masculine project of identity.

The musical elements themselves are, of course, evocative as sensibilia. The strummed instruments and the bass (or 'cello) provide the "metric pulse" of the music; a texture that has rhythmic and counter-rhythmic qualities that are interwoven and undulate. This texture, along with the vibrato cry of a viola, the shivering embellishments of a flute and the saccharine rubato of the vocals, affects what is referred to as *cengeng*, or the "weepy" quality of kroncong music (Yampolsky 1989: 6). This use of vibrato is akin to the *saudade* quality found in the Portuguese fado (Kornhauser 1978: 117). Vernon (1998: 3) remarks that there is no good translation of *saudade*, but refers to others who describe it as having a feeling of longing, nostalgia, yearning, piercing pangs of love, despair and sorrow. The term *fado* means fate, or destiny (ibid.: 2), and was used in the eighteenth century in the description of the Portuguese underclass as *fadistas*, or fatalists (ibid.: 6). Compared to the fado, the vocals and instrumentation of kroncong are produced with often "wider" and more "conspicuous" vibrati that, from my ear's perspective, edge towards an over-wrought, ostentatiously projected sense of yearning and melancholy (Kornhauser 1978: 143). The point is that in some instances, depending on lyrical content and context in which music is performed and heard, these musical elements attempt to evoke a sense of yearning and melancholy that are nostalgic, either in terms of a relationship, a moment in history or a place.

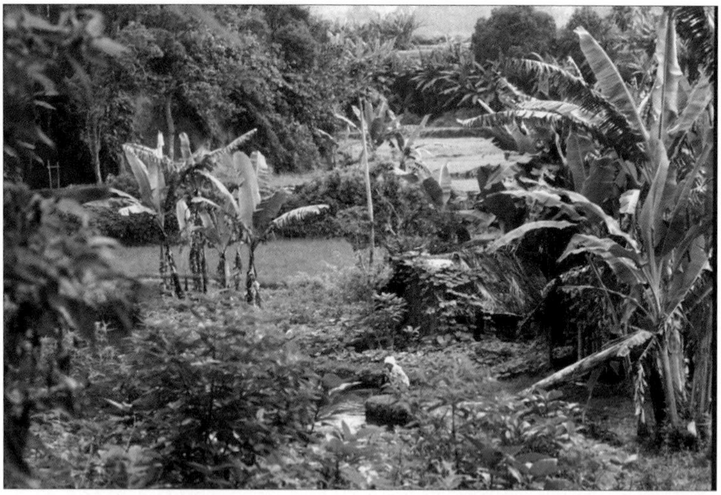

**Figure 2**
The "beautiful Indies" of Kroncong music. Photograph: Steve Ferzacca

During my time in Indonesia I encountered kroncong music in two places: in the kampung where I lived and at karaoke clubs. One afternoon, in a restaurant at a mountainside resort and hot springs in Bali, I watched a lone, middle-aged man in front of a karaoke machine singing the same kroncong song over and over. In the spirit of a particularly *modern* irony, here sat this man of the city in front of a big-screen TV with microphone in hand, dressed in the clothes of a businessman or *eksekutif*, surrounded by the remote mountain landscape of the Balinese countryside, looking at and singing to images of nature and the pastoral rusticity of village life. This mechanical reproduction of nature in a highly landscaped reproduction of nature – the resort – was striking.

As this moment of irony shows, the most obvious feature of kroncong is its "sense of place" (Feld and Basso 1996). While the repertoire is varied to include songs of romance (*romansa*), revolutionary songs (*kroncong revolusi*), nostalgic songs that yearn for the past, camp songs, songs that celebrate that afternoon leisure pastime of sociality known as *sore*, and recently updated pop music versions (*pop kroncong*), mostly about love or spousal relations, kroncong's sense of place is urban, even though its musical evocation includes songs for which a rustic lament replete with locally relevant metaphors from nature is often lyrically evoked. This may in part be the result of the gendered character of Age of Discovery European migrations. A mongrel mix of men as merchants, sailors, explorers and opportunists carried the fado genre for which romantic themes of love and heartbreak were the norm. Most likely, in the minds and mouths of men who circulated the Old World maritime trade networks that came to include the New World, the masculine lament was also for the pastoral, peasant countryside – but this is speculation indeed.

Tsuchiya (1989: 14) documents that in Indonesia kroncong, with its pastoral themes and imagery, converged with the appearance of a genre of landscape painting, originating with Dutch colonials and then taken on by Indonesian artists, that depicted the "beautiful Indies" with images of volcanoes and rivers, seas and coasts, rice fields and water buffalos, patches of bamboo and other tropical clichés. The "beautiful Indies" takes form in kroncong as a particular way of life, perhaps more importantly as a particular kind of society that in contemporary Indonesia is now said to be quickly disappearing in the face of development (*pembangunan*), modernization (*modernisasi*) and Westernization (*westernisasi*) – three historical processes that often are conflated. A nostalgia for the pastoral, rustic, village life is ever present in the "play of tropes" (Fernandez 1986: xiv) that characterizes the way many of my Javanese neighbors speak about urban life. Kroncong offers portraits of rural and urban lifestyles that have the capacity to function as meta-commentaries on everyday life in an urban kampung, or on the general state of affairs in what many see as a rapidly changing nation.

For example, a famous kroncong song, "Bengawan Solo" (Gesang 1940), tells the story of the Solo River. In the song lyrics the river represents the cycles of nature and the seasons, which for Java are the dry and wet seasons. The water of the Solo River is transmuted into human tears that are carried out to sea as a trader from the city of Solo (Surakarta) boards a ship. The sense of loss, longing and melancholy emerges from a play of temporalities that are represented as inherent to a place and form of social life. The city of Solo, the trader and the ship symbolize a temporality of movement and progress – life moving forward and away in time and space, leaving behind one lost in a pastoral paradise where time is cyclical, set to the rhythms of the seasons, and, therefore, predictable and unchanging. My friend, Pak Anu, owner of a small inn and son of a once successful batik factory owner, lamented the oncoming lifestyle of modernity and its sense of time. His remarks are typical, and reflect the spirit of kroncong's appeal.

> In the past the character of people and their lifestyle was different from today. A characteristic of people in Java at that time was patience. There were not as many people, and the land would grow anything people needed. All people had to do was wait and watch the rice, and the fruit trees, and the chickens grow, and then take what was needed; and rice, trees, and chickens would grow again. People were lazy. Today it's different [he pointed to his watch], people were not always watching the time. Time is different in the village, compared to the lifestyle of the city. Lifestyle is something new in Java. (Pak Anu, Yogyakarta, Indonesia – May 18, 1992)

Such commentaries commonly heard in local neighborhood debates juxtapose the unruly, continually changing heterogeneity of the modern city "lifestyle" with the predictable, determined traditional life found in the rustic countryside. Portraits of the countryside as nature and as a place of a particular social form with a set of social practices are simultaneously portraits of another place and way of life, in this case the city. Thus the nostalgia this musical genre evokes, the kroncong sense of place, is always double. Living in an urban kampung one always encounters this double sense of place as kampung residents attempt to reproduce village life in their own neighborhood settings. In general, *kehidupan kampung*, or kampung life, whether described in celebratory or in pejorative

**Figure 3**
Alleyways of Rumah Putri. Photograph: Steve Ferzacca

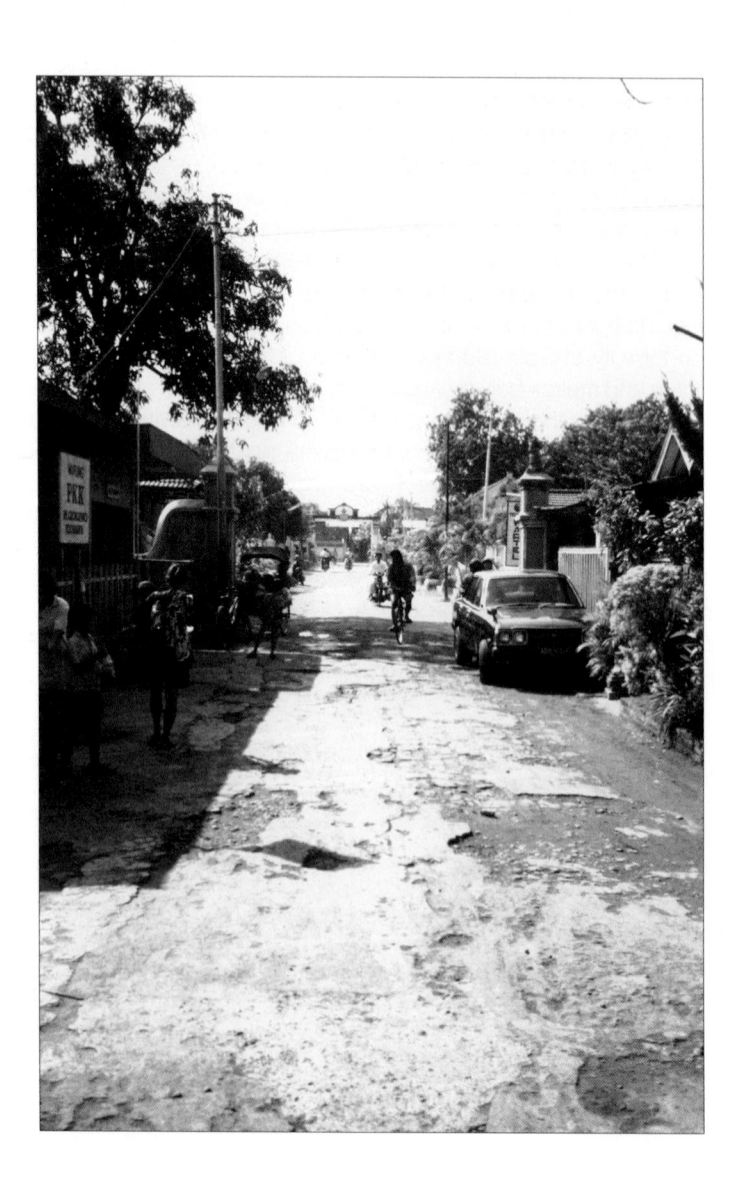

terms, is said to resemble village life (*kehidupan desa*). Features of both characterizations include closeness of social relations (if not density) together with reliance on social relations for making do and a common spirit of community, sentiments embodied in the Indonesian national emblem of cultural citizenship, *gotong royong*. But many will say that these features belong to a lost way of life found now only in the rural village, and existing only in fragments in the urban kampung. The *cengeng* sound conjoined with a social imaginary of the peasant countryside produces the affective charge of its nostalgia, and is a significantly shared kroncong sensibilia.

The kroncong sense of place as a "double-voiced discourse" (Bakhtin 1981: 325) for which the city and the countryside are continually in dialogue manifests the city as sensibly and sentimentally other. As discussed earlier, kroncong, like the trading port city, is an import. A long history of seas, lands and trade wind patterns not yet entirely overcome by advances in technologies of transportation ensured the establishment of trading port settlement communities in which emerged the urban kampung. The precolonial and colonial era kampung of trading port cities located in what is now Indonesia are described as more or less isolated living quarters where traders (often Malaysian but also other Southeast Asian ethnic groups as well as Chinese, Arab and Persian), lived, worked and worshiped.

The polyphony of kroncong sensibilia, sounded out in the musical elements, lyrical content and histories of making and listening to kroncong music provide a vantage point for cultural analysis, and, admittedly, much more could be made of these sensibilia in terms of cultural and social history than I have done so far. However, social structure is reflected in particular instances of making and listening to music as the sounds and sentiments judged worthy of expression, and therefore of remembering, are determined in a context of social relations. Making music, as one configuration of sound and sentiment within a particular community of social relations, takes place in a particular world of consequences: to make kroncong music in Rumah Putri, or any other kampung for that matter, is to engage in a social practice with some anticipatory response in mind. To put it another way, this act of sound and lyric possesses illocutionary force. In order to understand the communicative, and so practical, function of these kroncong rehearsals I ask that we look beyond the *apparent* referential qualities of kroncong sensibilia embodied in its musical elements, lyrics and topical themes. In order to get a sense of the force of making kroncong as a social practice I suggest we should consider this music's affective charge and indexical potentials as sensibilia that are not merely cultural in nature but have the potential to "move" people, and so operate as social forces. What I want to suggest here is that for the men who participated in the nightly rehearsals kroncong music embodies a particular range of Javanese masculinities, and so, in its production, allows for the possibility of their reproduction within the context of both "fantasized" and actual

Steve Ferzacca

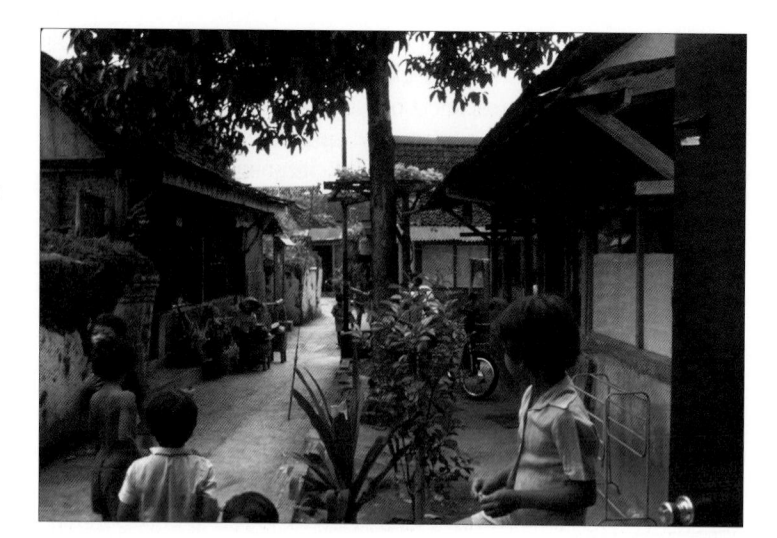

**Figure 4**
Kampung life. Photograph: Steve Ferzacca

Javanese gender relations. These "engendered and engendering" (Gutmann 1997: 834) possibilities are shot through with other forms of identity and consciousness that entangle class and ethnicity with gender.

### "Musicking" Social life in a Javanese Kampung

Situating kroncong's sounds and sentiments in the daily lives of people reveals not only the unexpected "diversions" and "trajectories" of a musical genre in various contexts (as a "social thing"; see Appadurai 1986: 3–63) but also illustrates how making music can be a tactical and strategic act, or as Herzfeld (1985: 25) puts it, an "agonistic display" in the poetics and politics of an ongoing set of social relations. Making kroncong music, then, is a cultural production within the real politik of community life – it is a "musicking" of social life, and in this kampung community this is a social life in which the shifting rhythms of gender relations can be heard. If our discussion of kroncong were only to touch on its sensiblilia of nostalgia, otherness, modernity, nationalism, and so forth found in its fields of representation we would miss the unexpected ways kroncong sensibilia are expressed and experienced, particularly within the dynamics of social relations.

However, there are many musics one encounters on a daily basis in the kampung. The bell percussions of gamelan are usually heard at special events like a wedding, at the Catholic church on Sundays, drifting through the air in the late afternoons from the small shadow puppet theater and with the lizard songs of the gecko from the all-night radio broadcasts of shadow puppet performances. Generational tastes in music shape these acoustic features of this soundscape. *Dangdut*, a music with influences from Middle Eastern music and South Asian film music, is frequently heard from radios and boom-boxes. Dangdut, often referred to as the music of the *rakyat* (people), has close associations with Islam, but it is generally the musical choice of the youth as dance music. Indonesian pop and international pop, rock and heavy metal music is coming both to influence and sometimes displace Dangdut as the youthful musics of choice, however (Wallach 2004). If the sounds of this built world of the kampung have something to do with social life, choosing a musical genre – like taking the decision to make kroncong music – is a choice in a "social poetics" (Herzfeld 1997: 15) for which locutions and hierarchy matter, but perhaps of a particular kind.

Rumah Putri is a self-aware, quintessentially Javanese kampung.[10] Classic styles of culture, or at least remnants of courtly airs and etiquette, are significant features of daily life in the kampung, and so are present in the social poetics of kampung life. As *Wong Jawa* (Javanese), Rumah Putri residents are particularly proud to be living on classic Javanese ground just outside the walls of the *kraton* (Javanese court) for which the city of Yogyakarta was founded. The value, and so appearance, that many of the kampung residents place on courtly postures and behaviors, the intentional use of Javanese language, particularly the emblematic use of speech registers, along with other classic Javanese cultural traits can at times make one feel as if one is living in "an antique land." This array of postures, gestures, linguistic and paralinguistic features are referred to by a variety of terms, but, in general, Rumah Putri residents say that one of the important markers of being a person the Javanese way is to be *sopan santun*, a term that includes these various behaviors with other social virtues (*budi pekerti*) for which the Javanese are famous throughout the archipelago. And while nothing of this has passed on without revision or reinvention, the gold standard for comparison of what is Javanese and what is not is often an aging list of *priyayi* (aristocratic) cultural traits, practices and values that mark an *alus*, or refined, cultured, sophisticated way of being-in-the-world. *Gamelan* music (*gendhing*), the music of the court, and the sound of alus, is certainly high on this list whether or not the Javanese actually listen to it (see Pemberton 1987). While it is often played by musicians of low social status from poor homes, *Gendhing Jawa* (Javanese gamelan) is one of the sensibilia of the *budi luhur*, or noble character, a relative status available to all, but, more often than not, possessed and nurtured by the courtly aristocrat. It was in this context that the kroncong rehearsals took place.

The rehearsals began after dark. They were loud affairs that lasted until midnight, and often later. The musicians assembled in front of the open door of a garage attached to Pak Wayang's house. Some of the neighborhood men (ranging in age from around 20 to 40) who often gathered at Pak Wayang's house participated in the kroncong rehearsals as singers in a kind of karaoke or open-mike approach to performance. For this reason they told me that they were rehearsing, and so making kroncong music as well – simply joining in designated them part of the "latihan" rehearsal, although basically they sat around and listened, played cards, drank a little bit, sometimes sang in the microphone. I could always count on finding this group of men smoking *kretek* cigarettes (clove), playing cards, talking and "searching for empty thoughts" (Ferzacca 2002) at Pak Wayang's house, kroncong rehearsals or not.

The audience, if that is what we can call that same small group of male onlookers and the passersby who would also stop and listen for a while, sat on the driveway inside the fence that surrounded his house, or on the porch of the house just off to the side of the driveway. Of course, in this tightly packed kampung we all became audience to these kroncong rehearsals whether we liked it or not. Pak Wayang's house was across the corner to mine, and all of the houses of the participants, except for the outsider musicians, were a stone's throw apart. On the occasions of the rehearsals the music could be heard well beyond our little corner of the kampung.

Except for the small group of men, my neighbors seemed to pay little attention to the music. The rehearsals did not draw a crowd. Excluding Pak Wayang and the musicians, the neighborhood men attending the rehearsals were related to each other either by blood or law. The majority of this group, except for Pak Wayang, were unemployed, underemployed husbands and youthful bachelors; I am unaware of the employment status of the musicians.

Pak Wayang, with his pencil-thin moustache, black leather coat, neatly pressed blue-jeans and established business with several motor vehicles, stood out in the context of the social relations and economic conditions of this corner of the kampung as a "visible sign" (Robison and Goodman 1996: 1) of prosperity and consumption. Pak Wayang, the sponsor of the kroncong rehearsals, is an entrepreneur who makes and sells hand-crafted *wayang* (shadow puppets) mostly to American and European tourists. At the time of the rehearsals he was, like myself, a new resident of this urban kampung; he had arrived only months before I rented our house in August of 1992. He had relocated his cottage industry wayang shop to this kampung because of its proximity to the *kraton*, the residence of one of two extant sultans, and because of the existence of a small and shabby, but well-known theater that hosts brief shadow-puppet performances in the afternoons. Pak Wayang's house, and so his shop, were a short distance from these tourist stops. He had been a rough-and-tumble, poor youth growing up in the streets of Yogyakarta. In the late 1960s and early 1970s, when this city and other parts of Indonesia were becoming known to a new kind of Western tourist globe-trotting on a shoe string, a certain degree of fluency in English had enabled him to work as a guide, attaching himself to them and showing them the sites in and around this classic Javanese city. This experience and his broken English, along with his continuing associations with foreigners and tourists, lent him a worldly, cosmopolitan air, which, because of his class background, were admired by some of the men and in the neighborhood. More importantly, Pak Wayang was a tangible example that such economic mobility could at least be imagined and possibly also attained. The men in the neighborhood were attracted to him for these reasons, but also because he provided opportunities for them to make small amounts of cash.

The choice to play kroncong music should be considered in the light both of the economic status of these men and other types of social status linked to peculiarly Javanese courtly social forms and practices as it may share certain aspects of Javanese language registers. The Javanese language is made up of several registers including a high register of honorifics (*krama*) and a lower register of speech used among intimates (*ngoko*). In the locutionary moment Javanese language registers are used to mark status differences among speakers and hearers. For the men gathered outside Pak Wayang's house, men of the "populist lower classes" (Robison 1996: 79–101 at 88), choosing gamelan music would constitute a speech act of sorts that would be similar to choosing to speak about oneself in high Javanese; a linguistic maneuver considered by the Javanese as always entirely inappropriate and especially so for men of this class. The choice to make kroncong music is the choice to use an orality of intimates, a low-register form of speech that is appropriate for public performance given these men's station in life.

Here we begin to see ways in which various forms of social hierarchy, past and present, fold into one another. The making of kroncong music in this working-class neighborhood represents a response to elite, aristocratic tastes in the cultivation of a populist cultural practice. The few extant social histories of kroncong music in Java agree that it developed in the "poorer quarters" of the cities in Java, was popular with Eurasians and other mestizo persons and was a musical genre associated with people of "questionable moral behavior" (Kornhauser 1978: 104). Because kroncong music played to a mestizo audience, in the context of Javanese society, for which the courtly arts and performance genres were the high-brow signs of a classic Javanese identity and a noble character, kroncong "had no authenticity" because it lacked a "classic style of culture" (Tsuchiya 1989: 19). It is important to remember that kroncong was bred in colonial context for which feudal social forms and practices were significant features of social life, not only among the Javanese but between the Javanese and the Dutch as well. In this context kroncong was to become the sound of an emerging Indonesian middle class (Yampolsky 1989: 10). More importantly, kroncong is a measurement and a chronicle; it is a sounding of a society increasingly organized by class rather than by rank and prestige of the court and its realm. Kroncong music traversed, over the course of history, the entire range of class boundaries as they were developing in Java and elsewhere in Indonesia. A music of the lower urban class, kroncong made its way up the ladder during the time of revolution and independence. As professional kroncong musicians emerged it became the music of the generation moving into adulthood (Yampolsky 1989: 12). As Yampolsky suggests, kroncong music, with the distinctive otherness projected by its "Western musical idiom and instrumentation" offered to this generation an "answer to the question of how to be modern" (ibid.:10) that was also a statement of how not to be modern; which by implication identified a classic style of culture.

However, these features of kroncong sensibilia were not those of greatest significance in the context of the nightly rehearsals on the porch of the house across they way. Neither were the men particularly interested in waxing nostalgic about the good old days or in romantic contemplation of pastoral village life. That said, in the context of other activities that were cover for carousing and drinking, for example over-night camping trips to the very places – the river, the mountain, the cave, the beach – that are imagined lyrically in kroncong music, I heard something of the "jargon of authenticity" (Adorno 1973) evoked lyrically and musically in kroncong sensibilia for the pastoral). Invitations to me to accompany them on these trips described the destinations as *masih asli*, or still authentic. Inferred in these invitations were opportunities to experience the pastoral as it once used to be for every Javanese but that now no longer exists except in remote areas of the countryside. I will never know if for the visiting musicians these feelings of melancholy and longing were aroused by making kroncong music. For the men of the neighborhood, however, making music was something else altogether. Making music those evenings, I contend, was about making gender through an expressive form that seeks recognition in the context of changing relationships between men and women in the kampung.

## Making Music, Gender Making

While other studies of kampung note class distinctions made among kampung residents that are derived spatially between those who live in the inner realm and those better-off residents who live along the outer streets, these distinctions in Rumah Putri did not seem significant in the daily lives of our neighbors. In terms of space what did matter, however, is the gendering of the kampung as "women's space." Murray (1991: 73, 84) also encountered an "internal community … culturally defined as women's space" for which matrifocality is the major pattern of residence and where the degree of mobility in and out of the kampung has come to define the public space of the kampung as domesticate, women's space in Jakarta. In Rumah Putri the cultural logic of kampung space and the social life that takes place within its bounds along gender lines have been re-shaped by the activities of the state-sponsored housewives organization that implements the government's health and development programs at the community level and by other similar programs in conjunction with the multiple-earning strategies often undertaken by women that are necessary for the social reproduction of family and community (see

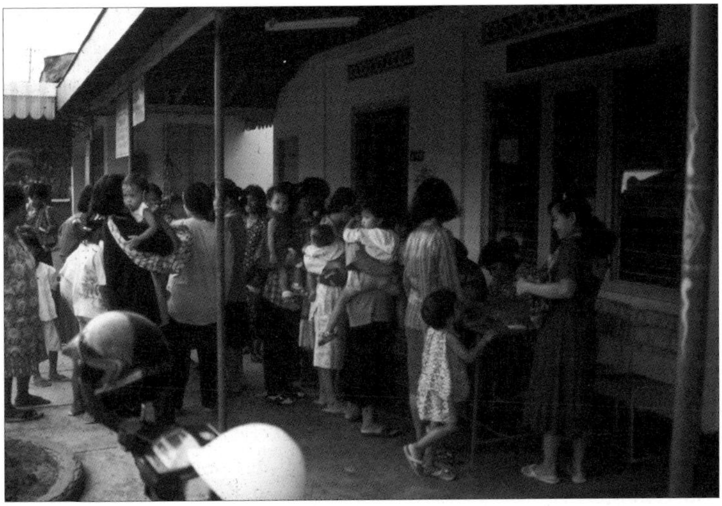

**Figure 5**
Extending domesticity in kampung space. Women weighing babies in the streets of Rumah Putri. Photograph: Steve Ferzacca

Newberry 1997). Recent productivity and policy shifts have placed an emphasis on women as stay-at-home mothers and community welfare workers (ibid.). As a result, the organization of kampung community and its maintenance fall more heavily on women. The community itself has become feminized in its reconstruction as a domestic community responsible for producing docile citizens and a ready, reserve army of labor.[11] One could extend the argument to suggest that the perennially underemployed men of the kampung find themselves living in an increasingly feminized social space.

The feminizing of public space in conjunction with consumption-based forms of status visible in the kampung, but also visible in the media, have had significant effects on gender relations in the kampung. Moreover, these aspects of social life are points with which men have had to contend in their constitutions of self and their projects of identity as men.

Years ago Michelle Rosaldo (1974), drew our attention to the relationships between the cultural construction of gender categories, the mobility of persons and the social use of space. She noted that among the Ilongot, the greater freedom of mobility for men relative to women was essential in defining "public" and "domestic" spheres of movement. In the case of this kampung, reproductive activities – the nurturing of family, care of home and of household finances – which were and are the responsibilities of Javanese women, have left the confines of home and become highly visible and public, both spatially and socially. The making of the home, through government sponsored development projects and the Pembinaan Kesejahteraan Keluarga – or Family Welfare Movement (PKK), has become the making of the community at large. While such dominance by women in the daily lives of men has been common inside the home, it is now out in the open. Whereas status and potency was once made evident by the numbers of people a man could draw around himself and his family at times of need, potency is becoming increasingly defined by the power to consume, rather than by retinues of people. At the same time women, through community development activities, revolving credit events and so forth, now have the capacity to mobilize numbers of people – mostly other women.

Other symptoms of this process in the "re-engendering" (Gutmann 1996: 834) of social space are apparent in the lackadaisical approach that those men who do hold the public administrative positions in our neighborhood group take towards fulfilling their obligations as community leaders, and the inappropriate kinds of work that the men say they desire given their class status, educational backgrounds, skills and training. In Rumah Putri, and in our neighborhood group, the male leaders, except for one or two, were mere hollow crowns of leadership and had very little to do with the decisions and activities needed to reproduce the kampung community. The person at the time responsible for the management of our municipally defined group of households never performed his duties and was rarely visible at municipal events in the neighborhood. On the other hand, a local revolutionary war hero acted as an elder and was called upon both publicly and privately (as we will see) in the ongoing formation of the community. Thus, in a sense, the domestic sphere, if such distinctions between domestic and public are still possible to make, completely engulfed the kampung space as women did the domestic work of the government in the reproduction of the community.

And many who study gender relations in Java would say this is typical. Men occupy legitimate positions of authority while backstage women make it all work. The conventional scholarly viewpoint on women and status in Java and elsewhere in Southeast Asia tends to highlight the "high status" of women, or at least the relative equality and complementarity of relations between men and women (Atkinson and Errington 1990; Jay 1969; Geertz 1961; Van Esterik 1982; see Peletz 1996 for a critique). While much of the ethnographic work on gender – and here the focus is nearly always women, although they are of course compared to men – interprets the prominence of women in the running of domestic affairs, management of household finances and in the markets (*pasar*) as evidence of the "astonishing degree of female dominance" in everyday life (Jay 1969: 92). Many ethnographic studies also point out the "disproportionate burden" placed on Javanese women (Jay 1969: 92; see also Geertz 1961; Newberry 1997; Wolf 1992). Others are quick to note as well that money in Java does not always equal power (Errington 1990; Keeler 1987; Wolf 1992).

Surprisingly, as far as gender is concerned, there is a paucity of focus on masculinity in the ethnographic record.[12] What we do hear of men is outlined, both from a scholarly and native point of view, in

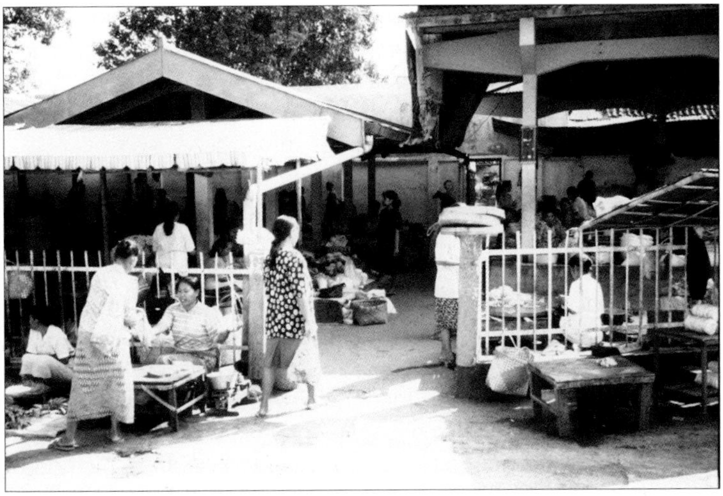

**Figure 6**
Women and the marketplace. Photograph: Steve Ferzacca

dualistic terms. In the little that exists on masculinity in Java, men are said to be "ideally" associated with potency and a concern for status, women with domesticity and money; men with the public sphere, women with the domestic; men with efficacy, women with diffidence; men with "reason" and order, women with "passion" and chaos. And the list goes on. Keeler (1990: 130) outlines the conventional understanding best: male qualities include "judiciousness, patience, self-control, deliberate speech, spiritual potency, a refined sensibility, insight and mystical capacity," while it is most probable that a female will be "emotional, crude, uncontrolled, uncontrollable, and likely to be ill-bred."

Brenner provides an interesting revision of sorts of these conventional representations and understandings of difference between the sexes, first by suggesting (correctly) that they represent elite *priyayi* ("aristocratic-cum-bureaucratic") gender ideologies that are now "commonly voiced among other elements of the Javanese population" (1995: 20–1). She goes on to locate "alternative" views by providing an account of the way in which "ideas about the human passions and the ability to control those passions" course through any supposed gender dualities in Java, and may in fact shape the practice of gender relations (ibid., p. 21). In her account, when Javanese men have money in their pockets they are at risk of losing control of their passions, spending money on prostitutes and gambling. Women, often characterized as more likely, compared to men, to lose control of their own passions, have the power, and so power (potency) as Javanese conceive of it, to control their husbands' passions by keeping hold of the purse strings. Rather than vulgar economic power, Javanese women practice a kind of asceticism by denying men something that has the potential to unleash their passions. Women, then, engage in a classic practice that is often only attributed to men as a way of obtaining and nurturing one's potency. With Brenner's alternate views I think we can gain a clearer sense of the role making kroncong music played in the gender relations of the kampung.

Through making music, Pak Wayang and the men attempt to address their increasing impotence as men in the affairs of kampung life. I realized this only in a moment of embarrassment. Often, Pak Wayang and the men chided me for not staying up all hours of the night – at least until the rehearsals had ended. I was told I was weak. As we sat and smoked cigarettes, listening to the kroncong, Pak Wayang remarked that making this music was an ascetic practice referred to as *prihatin*. The fact that the rehearsals lasted until well past midnight turned this leisure activity (*begadang* – staying up all night and talking) into asceticism (*melek*). It was, therefore, a method of developing and maintaining power. In fact, Pak Wayang and the men considered any activity that went on late into the night – gambling, camping trips, and making kroncong music – to be ascetic practice. The camping trips were described as rustic forms of asceticism: the men visited places traditionally considered ascetically potent – the same places nostalgically remembered in kroncong music – the river, the cave, the mountain. By contrast, women's mobility outside of kampung space is rather limited, especially after nightfall. The activity of over-night camping trips as male mobility and ascetic practice becomes linked to kroncong music as a particularly masculine mark of identity. Rather than showing nostalgia for the lost paradise of the pastoral, these men are nostalgic, it seems, for lost potency as Javanese men in the everyday social relations of the kampung.

While prihatin is not confined to men it is, nevertheless, considered an essential element in the making and enactment of social status (Anderson 1990 [1972] 17–77; Keeler 1987), and the locutions of public social status have generally been (for appearances sake), and continue to be, the concerns of men. Thus, prihatin is weighted as a male concern, as it is through men that women gain formal, public forms of social status. In this sense, leisure as prihatin is not merely a rationalization of play as something other than what it really is – rather, the conflation of leisure and ascetic practice points toward what I believe is the crux of the matter regarding the appearance of kroncong music in the kampung. If Keeler is correct, and I believe he is, that asceticism "offers an antidote to the corrosive capacity of interaction" (1987: 19), I contend that the conflation of leisure with asceticism begins to make sense vis-à-vis Brenner's (1995: 19–50) alternative view on Javanese gender identities. But first we need the final piece of this puzzle.

## The End of Kroncong

Of all the kroncong sensibilia one final one is worth mentioning and remembering, I think, from the point of view of Rumah Putri residents and those involved in making kroncong. In the early history of the Portuguese fado the fado musician was personified as a "drunk" or "tramp" (Vernon 1998: 2). Becker (1975) notes in her essay that before the professionalization of kroncong music kroncong musicians were often associated with a low-class masculine type characterized by unsettled mobility, uncontrolled sexuality and questionable moral character (see Lockhard 1998 as well). For kroncong, several metaphors capture the spectrum of this particular disposition of Javanese masculinities. In her brief but insightful essay on this "popular music," based mostly on Indonesian newspaper and magazine articles, she writes that early on kroncong became associated with "a Javanese stereotype known as the *buaya* (crocodile), or the *jago* (rooster)" (1975: 14). Both metaphors represent male gender possibilities for which swagger, danger and violence are significant terms. *Jago*, the low-register Javanese term for rooster, communicates the swagger quality of a Javanese machismo, and revolutionary heros are often referred to as jagos of Indonesian Independence. Indonesian Military personnel today are known for their rooster-like swagger.[13]

But it is the association of kroncong with dangerous marginal men, "ruffians" of questionable background and moral character, single, unsettled men, wandering the cities and countryside whose uncontrolled sexuality could unexpectedly and suddenly appear upon one's doorstep that stains this Javanese machismo as an unstable, menacing masculinity that is feared as much as it is admired. Frederick (1989: 251) describes the jago during the period of revolution and Independence in Indonesia as "uneducated, loosely principled kampung champions" who at the same time can also be described as "rural or merely petty criminal low-life." Kroncong music and musicians were historically exemplars of this nuance of Javanese masculinity. These wandering minstrels, referred to as *buaya*, were imagined to be villains, woman chasers, bullies and so forth who used kroncong music to seduce the "prostitute and the innocent maiden alike" (Kornhauser 1978: 129).

When the kroncong rehearsals suddenly ended the only explanation I was given by Pak Wayang and the men involved was that the rehearsals had become *bosan* (boring). If I had not been in the field with my wife, also an anthropologist, I mostly likely would have not become aware of events that led up to the end of kroncong in the kampung. An incident involving the husband of a women who lived next door to us illustrates the gendered tensions involved in making kroncong music, and supports Brenner's alternate view on gender relations in Java. This husband, chronically unemployed, was fond of the kroncong rehearsals: he would dress in his best blue jeans and silk shirt for them, and he told me that he planned to become a kroncong singing star. He had also been involved in an extramarital affair that had been discovered: at a public meeting the community had decided that he should cease the affair and return to his wife and family.

One evening this husband took money from his wife's purse for gambling and playing cards at Pak Wayang's house. Several of the neighbor women learned of this from his wife, and with the help of a respected male elder of the neighborhood (the war hero), Pak Wayang was told to stop the nightly card games that took place after the rehearsals. The gambling ended immediately. The women had come together, as they routinely do, to make community. The kroncong rehearsals ended shortly thereafter as well.

In addition, remember that Pak Wayang was, like us, a new resident to the kampung. He had moved there in search of a more profitable location for his puppet making enterprise, and he was quite successful as the ostentatious displays of his wealth and the flow of money made clear. As an outsider in this kampung of relatives he was always marginal, and the kinds of social activities he sponsored (gambling, disguised drinking, kroncong) were marginal as well as dangerous to the social fabric of the community. During our time in the field Pak Wayang diminished as a public figure in the neighborhood. His children, especially his daughters, stopped coming to our house to play with the other children, and his wife became increasingly isolated in her own home, so much so that the women of the neighborhood commented on her lack of presence, particularly at the women's community organization meetings. When I returned to Java Pak Wayang had moved from this neighborhood, his house remained empty as he searched for a tenant.

It is here that I want to consider the making of kroncong music as a "sign of recognition" (Keane 1997) that I see as a resounding recognition of *things as they are* as these men see it, and perhaps as they see themselves, and as they wish to see themselves given their particular social and cultural circumstances at the time. In terms of kroncong sensibilia, the buaya masculinity associated with making this music, a version of manhood perhaps more appropriate and available to lower-class men than the noble character of the refined aristocrat, was heard but unappreciated given the expectations of appropriate behavior in the neighborhood community managed in terms of gender relations. In the end, the men and their "passions" were kept in check; their invented ascetic disguises brought to light for what they really were: uncontrolled urges that Pak Wayang and the men had the audacity to display. The trangressive, even parodic attempts of the men to combine asceticism and potency of the Javanese noble character with the buaya virile, low-life character resounded by the rehearsals indicate creative, agentive attempts in a local project of identity. The kroncong rehearsals can be seen as a reflexive project of identity and a recognizably masculine sound that requires and expects a response "for its affirmation" (Keane 1997: 14) performed with a particular set of social relations in mind.

For those who made the music, the sensibilia of yearning and melancholy musically and lyrically central to kroncong music made sense, as Tsuchiya suggests, as a "longing for a place of rest and peace" (1989: 13–14) – a meditative response to the "all-over-present" (Geertz 1995: 138) of modern urban life. Kroncong's sense of place remains urban, and its timing modern, though the nostalgia for the pastoral, for lost love and so forth is forgotten in favor of a kind of "amnesia of anamnesis" (Casey 1987: 84), or forgetting to remember, rather than some longing for or memory of something lost. The attempt by Pak Wayang and the men to revise their rehearsals as ascetic practice, and their descriptions of them to me as attempts to search for "empty thoughts" – one of the goals of asceticism and the search for potency (see Ferzacca 2002) – should be seen in light of their social circumstances and the revisions to a cultural logic of place along gender lines. Making kroncong is a way of forgetting to remember, or perhaps forgetting to be aware of these circumstances, and perhaps this lends us an understanding of the sudden appearance and disappearance of the rehearsals. Thus, though the intent of kroncong sensibilia is to evoke nostalgia, yearning, and longing, for the Rumah Putri men kroncong music as a vehicle for such an experience was actually not all that nostalgic, nor a particular act-of-remembering.

It became clearer to me as I became attuned to the chords and discords of social life in the kampung that the appearance of kroncong music should be considered within the biographies of those involved, and the arrangements of those biographies as social relations. In expected and unexpected ways kroncong sensibilia go in and out of tune with the timbre and counterpoint of social relations particularly between men and women. As a "work of the imagination" (Appadurai 1996: 9) kroncong sensibilia that evoke urbanity, the pastoral, cosmopolitan modernity, nostalgic thought and so forth become sensible when in use as a "value-producing activity" (Marcus and Myers 1995: 4). I have tried to show here that making music is, as Schutz suggests, always a study in social relations. In some sense Pak Wayang failed in making social relations, but he and my neighbors, for a brief period, on those cool evening nights, did make kroncong.

## Notes

1. This research was supported by a Fulbright IIE Award (1991–2) and a Fulbright IIE Extension Award (1993). I should like to thank Lembaga Ilmu Pengetahuan Indonesia (LIPI) for their gracious support and help throughout the course of my project. I am particularly grateful to the American–Indonesian Exchange Foundation (AMINEF) who supported my research proposal and administered my Fulbright award. Thanks to Aaron Cox and Christine Yano who invited me to present this paper as part of a panel at a Society for Ethnomusicology Annual Meeting. I also

thank Andy Sutton for keeping me (and all those interested) well-informed on Indonesian musics and his mentorship on things Javanese. Perhaps most important, I should like to acknowledge Mbak Ning Raswani, Mbak Mei Sugiarti, Joan Suyenaga, Mas Hirdjan, Lani and Rio, Bu Yono, Bu Aseh, Mas Hendi, Pak Dimar, Pak Parno, Pak Edi, my other *kampung* neighbors, and all of the Yogyakarta residents I came to know for their assistance, intellectual input, but most of all for their friendship.

2. Schutz (1977) remarked that making music is a "study in social relations."
3. See also Abu-Lughod (1986) for a similar argument made a decade earlier than Roseman's.
4. Reference here is to Schieffelin's (1976) chapter on the ways in which song and oratory among the Bosavi of Papua New Guinea can "move people to tears." Since his work there is a voluminous literature in anthropology and ethnomusicology on the affective potentials of performance.
5. For an in-depth description of the musical qualities of kroncong music and its repertoire see Kornhauser's very fine essay (1978). In my brief descriptions here I often draw upon his musical terminology.
6. Again, for an excellent discussion of kroncong's historical relationship with the fado see Kornhauser (1978), but also see Harmunah (1987), Heins (1975), Kuntz (1973), Sumarsam (1992) and Tsuchiya (1989).
7. See Vernon (1998) for a history of the Portuguese fado.
8. Both Becker (1975) and Kornhauser (1978) point out that kroncong music after Independence became a "national music," and not a "nationalist" music, with little or no official support. Yampolsky (1989) lists kroncong along with bossa nova, dangdut and pop Indonesia as "national music genres."
9. See Sumarsam (1992), Lockhard (1998) and Yampolsky (1989, 1991) for a more complete and knowledgeable discussion of kroncong's history.
10. Rumah Putri is an overwhelmingly "Javanese" kampung. Newberry (1997), in her surveys of Rumah Putri and an enjoining kampung, noted only one person who was not ethnically Javanese.
11. See Newberry (1997) for an in-depth analysis of the political economy of labor and its gender implications in this kampung.
12. Of course Geertz's (1973) essay about Balinese men and their cocks is as much about masculinity as it is about status and cockfights. Peletz (1996) on gender in a Malay society is a well rounded study of gender with many excellent, in-depth discussions of Malay masculinities.
13. Kornhauser again describes how in colonial Batavia kroncong music was popular in the army camps (1978: 129).

## References

Abu-Lughod, Lila.1986. *Veiled Sentiments: Honor and Poetry in a Bedouin Society*. Berkeley: University of California Press.

Adorno, Theodor, W. 1973. *The Jargon of Authenticity*. Translated by Knut Tarnowski and Fredric Will. Evanston: Northwestern University Press.

Anderson, Benedict. 1990 [1972]. "The Idea of Power in Javanese Culture." In *Language and Power: Exploring Political Cultures in Indonesia*. Ithaca & London: Cornell University Press.

Appadurai, Arjun. 1986. Introduction: Commodities and the Politics of Value. In Arjun Appadurai (ed.), *The Social Life of Things: Commodities in Cultural Perspective*. Cambridge: Cambridge University Press.

—— 1996 *Modernity at large: Cultural Dimensions of Globalization*. Minneapolis; London: University of Minnesota Press.

Atkinson, Jane and Errington, Shelly (eds).1990. *Power and Difference: Gender in Island Southeast Asia*. Stanford: Stanford University Press.

Bakhtin, M.M.1981. *The Dialogic Imagination: Four Essays*. Michael Holquist, ed. Translated by Caryl and Michael Holquist. Austin: University of Texas Press.

Becker, Judith. 1975 "Kroncong, Indonesian Popular Music." *Asian Music* II(1): 14–32.

Brenner, Suzanne A. 1995. "Why Women Rule the Roost: Rethinking Javanese Ideologies of Gender and Self-Control." In *Bewitching Women, Pious Men: Gender and Body Politics in Southeast Asia*. Aihwa Ong and Michael G. Peletz, (eds), Berkeley: University of California Press.

Casey, Edward S. 1987. *Remembering: A Phenomenological Study*. Bloomington and Indianapolis: Indiana University Press.

Errington, Shelly. 1990. "Recasting Sex, Gender and Power: A Theoretical and Regional Overview." In Jane Monnig Atkinson and Shelly Errington (eds), *Power and Difference: Gender in Island Southeast Asia*. Stanford: Stanford University Press.

Feld, Steven. 1982. *Sound and Sentiment: Birds, Weeping, Poetics, and Song in Kaluli Expression*. Philadelphia: University of Pennsylvania Press.

Feld, Steven and Keith, H. Basso (eds).1996. *Senses of Place*. Santa Fe, NM: School of American Research Press.

Fernandez, James W. 1986. *Persuasions and Performances: The Play of Tropes in Culture*. Bloomington: Indiana University Press.

Ferzacca, Steve. 2002. "A Javanese Metropolis and Mental Life." *Ethos* 30(1/2): 95–112.

Frederick, William H. 1989. *Visions and Heat: The Making of the Indonesian Revolution*. Athens: Ohio University Press.

Geertz, Clifford.1973. "Deep Play: Notes on the Balinese Cockfight." In *The Interpretation of Cultures*. New York: Basic Books.

—— 1995. *After the Fact: Two Countries, Four Decades, One Anthropologist*. Cambridge: Harvard University Press.

Geertz, Hildred. 1961. *The Javanese Family: A Study of Kinship and Socialization*. The Free Press of Glencoe, Inc.

Gesang. 1940. *Bengwan Solo*.

Goldstein, Judith L. 1995. "The Female Aesthetic Community." In George E. Marcus and Fred R. Myers (eds), *The Traffic in Culture: Refiguring Art and Anthropology*. Berkeley: University of California Press.

Gutmann, Matthew C. 1996. *The Meaning of Macho: Being a Man in Mexico City*. Berkeley: University of California Press.

—— 1997 "The Ethnographic (G)Ambit: Women and the Negotiation of Masculinity in Mexico City." *American Ethnologist* 24(4): 833–55.

Harmunah. 1987. *Musik Keroncong: Sejarah, Gaya, dan Perkembangan*. Yogyakarta: Pusat Musik Liturgi.

Heins, Ernst. 1975. "Kroncong and Tanjidor: Two Cases of Urban Folk Music in Jakarta." *Asian Music* II(1): 20–7.

Herzfeld, Michael. 1985. *The Poetics of Manhood: Contest and Identity in a Cretan Mountain Village*. Princeton University Press.

—— 1997 *Cultural Intimacy: Social Poetics in the Nation-State*. New York: Routledge.

Jay, Robert. 1969. *Javanese Villagers: Social Relations in Rural Modjokuto*. Cambridge, MA: MIT Press.

Keane, Webb. 1997. *Signs of Recognition: Powers and Hazards of Representation in an Indonesian Society*. Berkeley: University of California Press.

Keeler, Ward. 1987. *Javanese Shadow Plays, Javanese Selves*. Princeton, NJ: Princeton University Press.

—— 1990 "Speaking of Gender in Java." In Jane Monnig Atkinson & Shelly Errington (eds), *Power and Difference: Gender in Island Southeast Asia*. Stanford: Stanford University Press.

Kopytoff, Igor. 1986. "The Cultural Biography of Things: Commodization as Process. In Arjun Appadurai (ed.), *The Social Life of Things: Commodities in Cultural Perspective*. Cambridge: Cambridge University Press: 64–94.

Kornhauser, Bronia. 1978. "In Defense of Kroncong." In Margaret J. Kartomi (ed.), *Studies in Indonesian Music*. Clayton, Vic: Centre of Southeast Asian Studies, Monash University.

Kunst, J. 1973. *Music in Java: Its History, Its Theory, and its Technique*. 3rd edn, Vol. 1., ed. E. L. Heins. The Hague: Martinus Nijhoff.

Lockhard, Craig A. 1998. *Dance of Life: Popular Music and Politics in Southeast Asia*. University of Hawai'i Press.

Marcus, George E. and Fred R. Myers. 1995. "The Traffic in Art and Culture: An Introduction." In George E. Marcus and Fred R. Myers (eds), *The Traffic in Culture: Refiguring Art and Anthropology*, Berkeley: University of California Press.

Murray, Alison J. 1991. *No Money, No Honey: A Study of Street Traders and Prostitutes in Jakarta*. Singapore; Oxford; New York: Oxford University Press.

Newberry, Janice. 1997. "Making Do in the Imagined Community: State Formation and Domesticity in Working Class Java." Ph.D. dissertation. Tucson, AZ: University of Arizona.

Peletz, Michael G. 1996. *Reason and Passion: Representations of Gender in a Malay Society*. Berkeley: University of California Press.

Pemberton, John. 1987. "Musical Politics in Central Java (Or How Not to Listen to a Javanese Gamelan)." *Indonesia*, 44: 17–29.

Robison, Richard, 1996. "The Middle Class and the Bourgeoisie in Indonesia." In In R. Robison and D.S.G. Goodman (eds), *The New Rich in Asia: Mobile Phones, McDonalds and Middle-Class Revolution*. London and New York: Routledge.

Robison, Richard and Goodman, David S. G. 1996. "The New Rich in Asia: Economic Development, Social Status and Political Consciousness." In R. Robison and D.S.G. Goodman (eds), *The New Rich in Asia: Mobile Phones, McDonalds and Middle-Class Revolution*, London and New York: Routledge.

Rosaldo, Michelle Zimbalist. 1974. "Woman, Culture, and Society: A Theoretical Overview." In M.Z. Rosaldo and L. Lamphere (eds), *Woman, Culture, and Society*. Stanford University Press.

Roseman, Marina. 1996 "'Pure Products Go Crazy': Rainforest Healing in a Nation-state." In Carol Laderman and Marina Roseman (eds), *The Performance of Healing*. New York: Routledge.

Schieffelin, Edward L. 1976. *The Sorrow of the Lonely and the Burning of the Dancers*. New York: St Martin's Press.

Schutz, Alfred. 1977. "Making Music Together: A Study in Social Relationships." In Janet L. Dolgin, David S. Kemnitzer, and David M. Schneider (eds), *Symbolic Anthropology: A Reader in the Study of Symbols and Meanings*. New York: Columbia University Press.

Small, Christopher. 1998. *Musicking: The Meaning of Performing and Listening*. Hanover, NH: University Press of New England.

Sumarsam. 1992. *Gamelan: Cultural Interaction and Musical Development in Central Java*. Chicago and London: University of Chicago Press.

Tsuchiya, Kenji. 1989. "Batavia in a Time of Transition." In Yoshihiro Tsubouchi (ed.), *The Formation of Urban Civilization in Southeast Asia*. Center for Southeast Asian Studies, Kyoto University.

Van Esterik, Penny. 1982. *Women of Southeast Asia*. Dekalb, IL: Center for Southeast Asian Studies, Northern Illinois University.

Vernon, Paul. 1998. *A History of the Portuguese Fado*. Aldershot: Ashgate.

Wallach, Jeremy W. 2004 "Dangdut Trendy: Is it Techno? Is it Traditional? No, it's Techno Hybrid Ethnic House Music." *Inside*

*Indonesia*, 78 (April-June). Available online at http://www.insideindonesia.org/ (accessed January 12 , 2005).

Wolf, Diane Lauren. 1992. *Factory Daughters: Gender, Household Dynamics, and Rural Industrialization in Java*. Berkeley: University of California Press.

Yampolsky, Philip.1989. "'Hati yang Laku,' An Indonesian Hit." *Indonesia*. 47: 1–17.

—— 1991 *Indonesian Popular Music: Kroncong, Dangdut and Langgam*. Music of Indonesia Series 2, Smithsonian/Folkways SF 40056, liner notes. CD-4735 v.2

# The Anti-Pod: After Michael Bull's "Iconic Designs: the Apple iPod"

## Kathleen Ferguson

Kathleen Ferguson is a Research Fellow in the New Learning Spaces project in the Faculty of Education, Monash University. Her research, including her Ph.D. "Sentient City," examines the ethics of sensory perception in modern metropolises.
Kathleen.Ferguson@Education.monash.edu.au

ABSTRACT   The branding of pleasure is ubiquitous, constituting one of those instances of modern life in which criticism seems humorless and heavy handed, while the ease with which consumer items insinuate themselves lightly suggests their being utterly innate. In this response to Michael Bull's warm reception of the iPod there is a sense of distrust at the emotional range the device (and its merchandising) engenders; it takes issue with the kinds of material and affective junctures that are called into being at the point at which the device stops being simply a tool for listening to music. What does it mean to tether one's enjoyment so firmly to a particular form or brand of product? By briefly raising Marx's work on the monetary economy and Adorno on the mass

**consumption of music, this review ponders whether there is room for both the social bond and the iPod in our pockets.**

> Everyone carries his social power, as well as the social bond, in his pocket (Karl Marx, *Grundrisse* 1973: 157)

Emotional responses are funny beasts; they pinprick rational responses and give us away, nowhere more so than when dealing with questions of the great secular spirituality of music: "my taste is good, your taste is not" would be the most likely equivalent of sectarianism. And now, with a new device to appreciate music, comes the possibility of reconfiguring all previous means of personalized listening with an ethos of infinite choice, incomparable mobility and ideal design. How could it help but draw out desires and expostulations? And so it seems that, whenever Apple's juggernaut media player is mentioned, there can only be a short window of time before the strong emotional response created by the machine is raised as a self evident feature that provides the *sine qua non* explanation for its popularity. Indeed, Michael Bull's defense of the iPod ("the supreme creation of an era") is well on the way towards lionizing the device, but doesn't touch on the complete market saturation of the product, so that similar alternatives are touted as "iPod Killers," the machines are common parlance among politicians and entertainers as a short-cut to cultural referencing and – beyond all else – the devices are seen as sufficiently valuable to steal, assault and even kill for.[1]

When we approach such hot topics in terms of cultural anthropology, we run the risk of being seen as "faddish," but the affective pull of such a domain leads us to a web of causations and consequence that is anything but *de mode*. For what is at issue are the techniques by which we may envelope ourselves in sensory experience as a way of counteracting the force of daily life. In the enactment of such a primordial need comes a welter of commercial and social transactions that step in to ameliorate isolation, boredom and the tyranny of "dead air" time. When a pleasure is presented as too insignificant a phenomenon to warrant serious critical investigation, that, itself, may be exactly the excuse for some kind of response.

Judging by previous work on personal stereo use (and by personal experience) it seems that such a device is used mainly in commuting, where the need for individualized pleasure if offset by the close proximity of others. At this stage, the phenomenon does not differ from previous forms of the same technology and it serves as a classic instance of human ability to soften the imperatives of labor, emotional detachment from the body and disenfranchisement from commonplace experience. I wish to argue that, if sensory experience is the point at which external input and internal consciousness collide to become *meaning*, then this is a process that needs to be analyzed, exercised and subjected as much as possible to a kind of ascesis of sensual awareness. While Marx talks about this emancipation of the human senses as leading to the overcoming of private property, the desire for sense-based self-knowledge in this paper is far more pedestrian. But still, there is a particularly charismatic challenge that is offered by the young Marx – to affirm the value of each tool of daily use in such a way that we see it for its usefulness, its beauty, its capacity for affect in a way that is critically aware of the powerful mediating forces at work between ourselves and the products we buy. A contemporary reading of such a project may mean we are free to continue with our examined lives – without the hair shirt.

While it may belabor Marx, it should be noted that the Barthesian link between the DS Citroën and the Gothic cathedrals (and, by inference, the iPod) does draw these three phenomena towards the misty, opiate infused realm of the sacral. And while the link between the flying buttresses of Christendom and a luxury sedan may be ingenious, the connection between those same sacred spaces and the minute world of the personal stereo is not unknown. In a presentation entitled "Some Thoughts on Ringing" Judith Williamson – whose 1986 essay providing one of the earliest critiques of the Walkman in English, "Urban Spaceman," is a foundation text on many a cultural studies course – makes much the same point. She notes,

> around the whole world, the bell was absolutely central as a one form of communication within a community. The ringing of a church bell, or the bell of a Mosque or a tower is the one sound that can be heard ... it seems to me that the Walkman is the exact antithesis, it's actually being in a public space and having a sound in your ears that nobody else can hear apart from you. (Williamson, 2003)

For Williamson, as for Bull, sound is constitutive of space. And, in this case, it appears that social space is receding from peeling countryside or the Bow bells, to the microcosm of an ear canal. This shrinking calls to mind the monetary economy as it is defined by Marx. As the value of commodities is jettisoned from their use value, to take on symbolic meaning, so too are social relations atomized – suggestive of their being secreted away in back pockets and stored away for a moment best fitting expenditure. Certainly, the argument for the ever decreasing scale of consumer icon is convincing, so that the apex of culture shrinks from Rouen cathedral, to *le goddess*, to a mobile stereo, but there is something about this sense of enchantment that feels like a slippage here. Where consumers speak of the tactile qualities of their purchase - "It feels good to hold it in your hand, to rub your thumb over the navigation wheel and touch the smooth white surface" - as a typical response (in Bull, 2006), they remain strangely silent on what you might imagine was the primary purpose of the product: to play music. As a secondary consideration, the mobility and personal choice of music becomes an issue, but there is a somewhat synesthetic response to the iPod that comprehends it as much in terms of touch and vision as sound. The splitting of purpose from value is telling, it provides the originary moment of the fetishized commodity, and the moment at which this break is made may, I hope, give some indication of the significance behind the fetish – what it is that we hope for when we carry white cords from our eardrums.

## The Sound of White

There is a quasi-religious underpinning to the tactile delights that are mentioned by Bull's iPod users: "It's almost as if my iPod understands me" is a refrain that clearly wishes to go beyond Marshall McLuhan's suggestion of technology being an extension of our senses. This scenario would be relatively naturalized, in comparison with the machine that knows us better than we know ourselves. This projection of all our needs and desires is ennobled through tools much greater, or at least more aesthetically pleasing, than the flawed mental and physical capacities of our selves, now seemingly inadequate to the task of living. In their place are machines that offer a model of an ideal self we could never be, a streamlined entity with preternatural instinct for coping with an environment that is comparatively underwhelming. The "shuffle" function speaks of an intuitive machine where the ability to replay tunes in random order is interpreted with a very human wish for significance. It is seen as a message, a moment of telepathy between user and machine that is not shared with the world, but which reflects upon it, framing it with aural ambience. Machine and user are perfectly suited. This is a transcendent point, where the quotidian acts of commuting, walking, performing menial tasks, are illuminated and made into something else. Certainly, this function is not singular to Apple's media player, indeed it is the locus of all personal stereos. Instead it is the appearance of the iPod, its size and its blank, white skin, that has it seated in the pantheon of retail icons.

Whiteness was not the domain of personal electronic goods before 1999: it was the color of refrigerators and washing machines. When it came to be associated also with the Apple Mackintosh range of computers, it ushered in a harnessing of affect that marketers could only have dreamed of – while the shape and scale of the products was not always widely accepted, the color (a neutered shade of white that echoed operating theaters, industrial kitchens or the blizzard of white-on-white themed apartments that appeared in interior design magazines) that clearly caught the social imagination. Perhaps this is not the time to ponder on just what happened to engender a shift towards "the clinic" in Western culture, but I'd like to at least moot it as a phenomenon located in a particular place and time that had its effect in a high degree of permeability between the corporate/social imaginary and the personal/ individual, which reminds me of the success of cigarettes in the 1940s and 1950s. Or more so, for, stepping aside from the deleterious effects of smoking, the all-pervasive sense of glamour had to be inculcated through endless Hollywood films before reaching the level of public consciousness that it did. Instead, with a relatively small but iconic print advertising campaign, focused primarily on billboards in public spaces, the iPod achieved a level of brand recognition that resulted in a large market and an even larger sphere of influence. Like "Kleenex" and "Hoover" in their own markets, the brand of this product has come to stand for the general category of personal media players – this is no doubt largely due to its phonetic simplicity, but it remains the singular point to which a complex chain of signification is tethered. Forty-two million products sold in under five years suggests that whatever is signified relates to some alchemical combination of desire and uncertainty that emits a siren call.

Of course, in international commerce, nothing – color, shape, design - is arbitrary. The iPod, if not white, is likely to be pastel pink, green or blue. It is flat, its edges rounded, its tuning device is large and central – it is form honed to its clearest function. It is a far from instinctual process, to reconfigure music into bits and memory that can be stored, ripped and burnt, but this is made palatable by an "interface" that all but commands your action and imperceptibly moves you towards a single vendor of pre-packaged digital music (Apple's own internet-based media "store"). Over one billion tunes and 15 million movies downloaded in five years suggests the nexus between each little plastic unit and the mother-ship is secure. (Gilbert, 2006) The tactile encounter with the product may be the one that is most often mentioned in reviews, but the iconic advertising and somewhat staged performance of wearing the device – not to be tucked into any pocket, although this is simply a personal observation – suggests that the pleasure is one of managed social stratification. There is the pleasure of similarity with an advertised ideal of silhouetted hipsters, as well as with fellow consumers, and there is the delight of difference, always a part of personal stereo use and particularly obvious in the display of status through commercial brands. Is it this that tugs at our heart strings and renders us less interested in the sound to be heard therein, than in the touch, the visual display and the kinesthetic satisfaction of a body in sync with the normative values of late Capitalism?

## Arming the Affective Body

As critics of a sensory bent, there are particular questions about the way not simply our emotional range, but the very thresholds of our bodies are targeted in ways that are both nuanced and interpellative – not least in the way we are called to listen to music in a certain way; self-consciously, in a privatized public state of bliss. As a result, this requires a line of inquiry that does not switch off at the end of the working day, but continues to track the commercialization of affect beyond the stage where it can claim to be "natural," to hunt down the processes that engineer our needs, our sense of inadequacy, our preference for delegating unpleasant emotional tasks to the machines that were meant simply to be their conduit. And then what? This may be an end in itself. This is the prospect that Adorno raises in his essay on the function of music and, correspondingly, the criticism of music as a means of "obtaining a concept of society through one's own sensorium." Ultimately it may be enough simply to, "without harbouring any illusions about the outcome[,] … say what (you) know" (Adorno, 1976: 39–54 at 54). In this regard, the senses are politicized (again?) as the internalized site that we carry around and through which we know the world. But such a project would be loaded with the imperative of our physiology, as well as its perviousness to the affective manipulation of advertising. It may be that such a process leads on to a process of engagement that precedes the cultural, political and economic realm – a form of sensory citizenship in which franchise is nothing more (and nothing less) than our sentient bodies.

## Note

1. On April 23, 2006, Belgian teenager Joe Van Holsbeeck was killed in central Brussels after refusing to give his MP3 player to thieves. The brand of player has not been mentioned in any of the media reports, anywhere. This compares with a report from New York that only the Apple products are generally targeted by thieves, with other brands being seen as insufficiently desirable to enter to illicit economy.

## References

Adorno, Theodor. 1978/99. *Sound Figures*. Stanford: Stanford University Press.

———.1976. "Function." In *Introduction to the Sociology of Music* New York: The Seabury Press.

Bull, Michael. 2006. "Iconic Designs: the Apple iPod." *Senses and Society* 1 (1): 105–9.

Bull, Michael and Back, Les (eds). 2003. *The Auditory Culture Reader*. Oxford: Berg.

Feuerbach, Ludwig. 1972. *The Fiery Brook; Selected Writings of Ludwig Feuerbach*. Edited by Z. Hanfi. Garden City, New York: Anchor Books.

Gilbert, Mark. 2006. *Apple Should Succumb to IPod Porn Temptations*. Available online: http://quote.bloomberg.com/apps/news?pid=10000039&cid=gilbert&sid=atmv9JE0pOIQ] (accessed May 4, 2006; last viewed April, 11, 2006).

Hamilton, Clive. 2006. "The Death of Social Democracy." *Quarterly Essay* 21 (1): 1–70.

Marx, Karl .1967. "Feuerbachian Criticism of Hegel." In *Writings of the Young Marx on Philosophy and Society*. Edited by L. D. Easton, K. H. Guddat. Garden City, New York: Anchor Books.
——. 1974. *Grundrisse - Foundations of the Critique of Political Economy*. Harmondsworth: Penguin
Williamson, Judith. 2003. *Some thoughts about Ringing*. Available online: www.slowfall.org/pages/talk3.php (accessed October 13, 2005).

# Cultural Politics

**Edited by John Armitage**, University of Northumbria,
**Douglas Kellner**, University of California, Los Angeles and
**Ryan Bishop**, National University of Singapore.

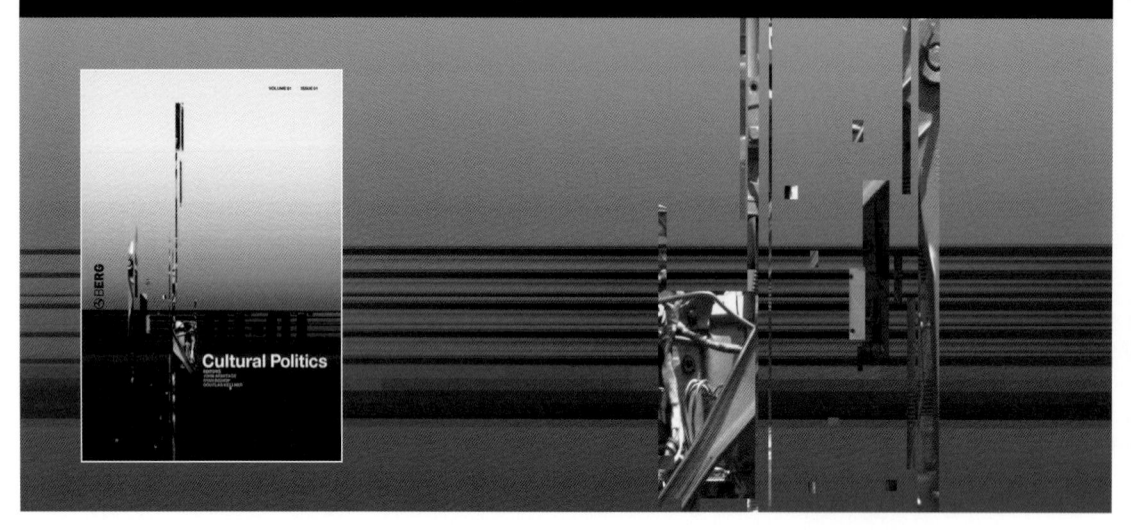

***Cultural Politics* explores precisely what is cultural about politics and what is political about culture.**

*Cultural Politics* publishes work that analyses how cultural identities, agencies and actors, political issues and conflicts, and global media are linked, characterized, examined and resolved.

While embodying the interdisciplinary and discursive critical spirit of contemporary cultural studies, this journal also emphasizes how cultural theories and practices intersect with and elucidate analyses of political power.

### Board members include:
Paul Virilio, Gayatri Chakravorty Spivak,
Nigel Thrift and Chua Beng Huat.

**Indexed by:**
IBSS (International Bibliography of Social Sciences), SocINDEX (Ebsco) British Humanities Index, Sociological Abstracts and Political Science Abstracts (CSA).

Published 3 times a year in March, July and November.

| ISSN: 1743-2197 | Individual | Institutional |
|---|---|---|
| 1-year subscription 2006 | £40/$75 | £155/$279 |

**BERG**

Order online at www.bergpublishers.com or call +44(0)1767 604951
Institutional subscriptions include online access through www.IngentaConnect.com
To order a sample copy please contact enquiry@bergpublishers.com
View issue 1.1 free online at www.ingentaconnect.com

**Sensory Design**

# Restorative Bath Waters: Bath Spa, Bath, England

## Christie Pearson

> The Most Sovereign Restorative BATH WATERS Wonderful and most excellent agaynst all diseases of the body proceeding of a MOIST CAUSE as Rhumes, Agues, Lethargies, Apoplexies, The Scratch, Inflammation of the Fits, hectic flushes, Pockes, deafness, forgetfulness, shakings and WEAKNESS of any Member Approved by authorite, confirmed by Reason and daily tried by experience.
>
> Early enticement to bathe in Bath

Christie Pearson is a writer, artist, architect and co-director of the WADE festival of performance and installation art in Toronto's wading pools (www.wadetoronto.com). She is writing a book on bathing.

The new Bath Spa in Bath, England, elegantly continues an exploration thousands of years old on this site: how to connect ourselves with each other, the land and the cosmos through ritual and building. In 1997 the Millenium Fund supported the region's proposal to have access once more to Britain's only naturally-occurring thermal springs, flowing down the sewer for the last thirty years. While the spa, as a concept and an architectural type, is at the forefront of contemporary taste and preoccupations the roots of Bath as a center of bathing reach far into antiquity.

Here, in the Roman Bath Museum, I lean over a seventeenth-century balustrade to look down into the murky aqua waters of the King's Pool, which once served a monastery-run hospital. Down below are Roman foundation walls, built to enclose a natural sacred spring of the Celts. The first-century Roman sanctuary precinct of Aquae Sulis was organized along the axis of the spring, the sacrificial altar and the temple of Sulis Minerva, whose name shows the Roman usurpation of a Celtic deity's power. Continuing an 8,000-year tradition of human occupation, Roman soldiers and statesmen would come to repose, heal and make offerings to the spring's deity.

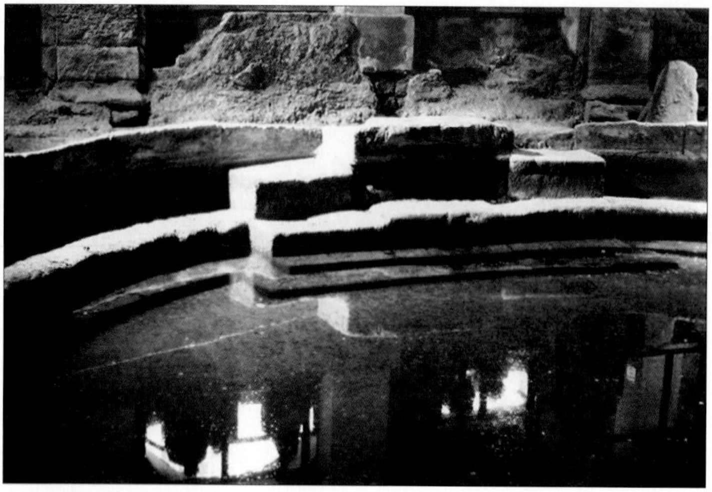

**Figure 1**
Second-century cold plunge pool, Roman bath complex, Roman Bath Museum. Photograph by Christie Pearson.

While hygiene concerns ended Roman-themed bathing parties in the King's Bath in 1978, the heyday of Bath as a spa ended in the 1930s. A visitor of the early century could repair to the Cross Bath, the Hetling Baths, the Royal Swimming Bath, the Tepid Swimming Bath, the Royal Baths, the Queen's Baths, or the King's Bath and Hotspring amidst a busy tour of site-seeing. Victorian hygienic fads and water cures are our culture's most recent tradition of "sanitum per aqum." Stainless implements, nozzles, hoses, grab bars and bleached uniforms that we can find in European spas can strike our post-industrial sensibilities as comical. The Dutch Thermae Development Company think we have an appetite for something else.

The new Bath Spa features an ambitious program of new construction combined with historical restoration of five buildings, all in the core of historical Bath. The Hot Bath, built in 1773, is incorporated into the new spa, negotiating its volume with the city. The architect of the Hot Bath, John Wood, and his father helped make Bath the epitome of Georgian style and the ideal resort town. It now holds twelve treatment rooms for alternative preventative and curative therapies. A reassuring weight of stone tightly encloses a deep pool, offering both grounding and suspension. Looking up I continue to float through a finely engineered glass roof.

Set apart from the rest of the complex is the Cross Bath, a designated historical building and sacred site, a small folly into which only a few bathers are allowed at a time. The interior of the court gives you an oval portrait frame to the sky, whose moods and faces will become visible as you start to melt in the 45°C heat of the water which rises directly from one of the three sources below.

The new building is designed by Nicholas Grimshaw and Partners (whose Eden Project also reflects an eco-technological utopian vision) with structural engineers Ove Arup and consulting architect Donald Insall Associates. The product of this association is a design at once energy-efficient and playful: a glass wrap enclosing a cube of local limestone formally refers to the historical buildings that have now become wrapped into the ensemble. It minimizes carbon dioxide and heat loss, uses low-emissivity glass and strategically captures and holds solar energy in its envelope. Thermal spring water also heats the building and preheats shower and washing water. All baths use spring water, filtered through a natural sand system and treated with earth-friendly ozone water purification.

The large thermal swimming pool is half-sunken below street level, amplifying the sense of immersion into the layered ground of the city. Columns emerge from the water drawing the eye up to curve across the flare and return down, Gothic allusions tracing a grotto's branching canopy.

Beneath me a weighty foundation requires nearly two hundred piles to support a meter-thick slab and tons of mechanical equipment. Here, the steamy water is cooled to 35°C for swimming. Bath's thermal water is 10,000 year-old rainfall, heated 2 km below the earth's surface and forced back up through a fault to emerge beneath the Roman Bath, the Cross Bath and, now, to feed the new spa. Significant amounts of sulphate, sodium, calcium chloride, bicarbonate, magnesium, silicon and iron will draw people with stress, muscular-skeletal, post-stroke and injury, sports rehab and cardio-respiratory ailments as well as those with a love of sensual pleasure.

Bath water's skin-healing properties are recorded in the legend of prince Bladud, who returned from his education abroad with leprosy. Disguised as a swineherd, he imitated his pigs and healed his wounds in the muddy waters. The story relates to annual renewal and rebirth in the earth and the theme of the ailing solar king who is rejuvenated by the lunar-female element. I recall the pair of Sol and Luna friezes in the museum. Is our collective fatigue from solar positivism spurring the current spa revival?

After my earth immersion in the pool, I climb stairs lined with porthole views to the shrinking city. Open floors house solitary and collective pods: first wet, where frosted glass cylinders lit from below enclose steam rooms and showers; then dry, for massage, physiotherapy, nutrition and classes. I then emerge to the light of day or the black of night to a rooftop pool overlooking the surrounding hills. Not shying from the symbolism of enacting an archetypal voyage, this spa differs from the Victorian model as it addresses me as a sensual, emotional, intellectual and spiritual being. I experience the elements composing my body, the building, and the broader ecological networks and movements in our collective building culture.

# The LDS Conference Center

## William C. Miller, FAIA and Ryan E. Smith

### The Gentile's Perspective

William Miller and Ryan Smith are faculty members in the College of Architecture + Planning at the University of Utah in Salt Lake City. Professor Miller (the "gentile" – non-Mormon) is the former Dean of the College, and, while not a member of the LDS church, he finds the connections between architectural form and religion an intriguing study. Assistant Professor Smith (the "saint") is a member of the LDS church and has attended various events at the Conference Center. He has never realized the impact of the religion on his aesthetic tendencies until critically writing this review. miller@arch.utah.edu

When I was growing up in the West, Salt Lake City was considered a "peculiar place," as the City of the Saints appears rooted in a unique world-view and resulting physical order. In the process of moving to Salt Lake City over a dozen years ago, my two sons asked our real estate agent what living in the city was like – her response set a stage for understanding the place that continues to inform me today. "You must remember," she said, "that Salt Lake City is an orthodox community, which creates a unique condition that few in this country, or the western world, experience."

Founded in 1847, Salt Lake City was platted as the "City of Zion" by Brigham Young. This act had great impact on the physical structure of the city. With ten acre, 640-foot square, city blocks, intended to be parceled out to maximize an agrarian vision of land use and habitation – and 100-foot street right-of-ways, to allow a six-oxen team wagon to do a U-turn in the street – the spatial structure of Salt Lake City is profoundly different than her western American counterparts. These large blocks and wide streets provide a spacious sensation as one transverses the city, while simultaneously, gathering in dynamic, panoramic views of the Wasatch mountain range. Further, there is a much less dense urban fabric than found in her sister cities, due to the building patterns imposed by the large blocks. And the city contains the navel of the Mormon universe: Temple Square, the spiritual center and home of The Church of Jesus Christ of Latter-day Saints (LDS).

This religious center impacts the city profoundly: First, the streets are numbered sequentially from Temple Square toward the four cardinal points; that is 100 North, 100 South, 100 East and 100 West and so forth. Given the coordinates of my address, for instance, it means I live nine blocks south and twelve blocks east of the Square. Moving through the city, one is palpably aware of the streets' relationship to the Square, as the coordinate system constantly articulates one's position within the city as well as the entire Salt Lake Valley. Second, the Square holds two of the most important architectural works of the LDS faith – the Salt Lake Temple and the famed Tabernacle.

Therefore, when, in the mid-1990s, the church decided to build the Conference Center, it was an act whose significance cannot be overstated.[1] First, to address the current and future needs of the church, it would replace the 6,000-seat Tabernacle used for the church's biannual General Conferences; second, it acknowledged the important position that the LDS church has assumed in the recent past within the world community of churches; third, from an outsider's perspective, it appears the most significant architectural undertaking by the church since construction of the Salt Lake Temple and Tabernacle; and, last, at 1.4 million square feet, 9.43 million cubic feet – filling one ten-acre block – it would have a very significant presence in the fabric of downtown Salt Lake City.

The building steps up, and out of the block-square site as a large, terraced granite mesa, surmounted by an alpine roof garden. The roof garden provides a counterpoint to Temple Square, which it overlooks. As a center of spirituality, the Square is a landscaped oasis and haven walled from the profane city. The roof terrace provides a second center, with the sensation of being on a mountain that provides an awe-inspiring prospect to the Valley of the Saints. And, unlike the protected garden below, the mountaintop is windy and sunny, bearing the full impact of the high- desert environment. Against the sound of the wind blowing through trees and grasses in the background, the sound of water emanates from the fountain in the center of the mesa. The fountain metaphorically issues, as the streams form in the mountains surrounding the city to send life-giving water to the valley. The fountain cascades down the front of the complex and joins the recreated City Creek Canyon waterway at the edge of the entry plaza. Oasis and mountain, two essential places in the desert: one offering protection while the other provides the resources necessary for dwelling.

The terraced massing, combined with the giant staircase and waterfall cascading down the front of the complex, appears at one

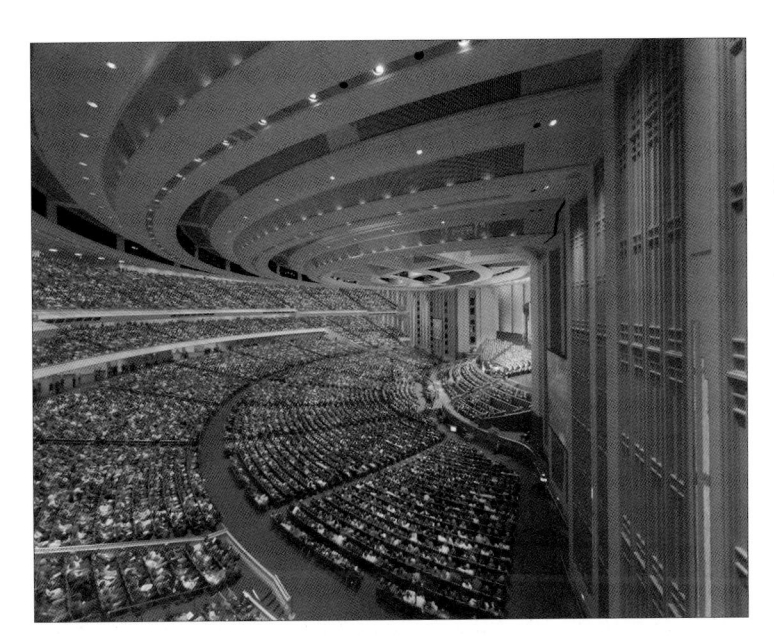

**Figure 1**
The Filled Assembly
Hall during Conference.
Photograph:
Timothy Hursley.

level like a monumental village positioned on the large entry plaza. Yet the large planar granite surfaces simultaneously provide a modernist appearance. Waggishly referred to as the "Supernacle", the exterior evokes a variety of images and associations – from Pre-Columbian to Babylonian, and even a bit of Albert Speer. The cool, smoothly hewn granite cladding of the complex was taken from the same quarry used to finish the Salt Lake Temple over a century ago, providing a tactile, visual and spiritual connection between the two works. The one element providing an obvious sense of religiosity, the tower over the waterfall, was added late in the design process and is less than convincing within the overall composition.

Among the largest theater-style buildings in the world, the center is the premier meeting hall for the LDS church, seating over 21,000 individuals in a column-free, fan-shaped auditorium. Prophetic speech-making, dramatic performances, elaborate reenactments of scripture and congregational educational activities are at the heart of Mormon culture, so within this tradition the Conference Center acts as the symbolic stage for this growing international religious culture. The interior space is stately, yet the cavernous size of the grand circulation hall and auditorium gives the impression that it can easily swallow up its 21,000 attendees. Illuminating the sheer magnitude of the space, the auditorium could, theoretically, hold a Boeing 747 within its walls. When it is empty, the sheer volume of this impressive space forms a palpable auditory silence.

## The Saint's Perspective

Temple Square in Salt Lake City is the preeminent pilgrimage site for the international membership of the Church of Jesus Christ of

Latter-day Saints, commonly referred to as the Mormons. Saints travel from around the world to attend bi-annual church conferences at the center and view the neighboring iconic and historic Temple and Tabernacle. Announcing plans to build the Conference Center in 1996, LDS church President Gordon B. Hinckley stated that it was conceived out of recognition that the Tabernacle no longer held all those who desired to attend conference. In addition, the new Conference Center, with its mountain-like presence within the city and international broadcasting power was to stand as a symbol of worldwide faith.

The church describes its mission as "the fountain from which truth rolls forth to fill the earth."[2] Water plays an important religious role through ordinances (which are like sacraments) such as baptism, and it stands as a symbol of Christ to which members look for spiritual cleansing and nourishment. Fountains can be found throughout the complex. First, at the level of the street facing Temple Square on the south side, water separates the plaza from the street and flows westward along the natural slope of the valley floor. The sound and image of water greets visitors again within the building where a waterfall formed from two joined roof-garden fountains cascades down, mediating between the viewer and the exterior plaza. Reminiscent of the flowing creeks and rivers in nearby canyons feeding the Great Salt Lake, the sensory experience of the flowing water is visual, auditory and tactile. Breezes from adjacent City Creek Canyon waft down through the valley and into the downtown. These moderate winds frequently cause water from the cascading fountain to lightly spray conference attendees as they are circulating up, around and outside the building.

The ascent and descent of people on the exterior and interior of the building along stairs, escalators and broad corridors, coupled with the culminating, spectacular view from the top of the roof gardens, suggest the notion of a far reaching, expanding, worldwide church. For those attending a church conference the sequence of spaces is experienced in four stages: the exterior plaza, the grand interior circulation halls, the auditorium and the exterior terraces and stairs (including the roof garden). First, the act of gathering at the entry street-level plaza space – despite the number of people present – organizes individuals into orderly lines through specific access portals. While initially sensing one's aloneness in this sea of international attendees, the sequence gradually becomes more intimate as the experience moves into the building. With anxious anticipation, visitors ascend on escalators within the mountain-like building to the various levels of the grand, multi-tiered circulation hall. In the impressive interior hall an original glass sculpture is sited under a skylight connected to the tower, spatially connecting the roof garden to a floor fountain in a continuous vertical space. The circulation halls also serve as a church art museum, containing some of the most identifiable paintings in the church's short history in addition to housing many contemporary paintings and sculpture depicting religious themes. The top-floor circulation hall offers a space of particular impact where a stunning view of the Temple is framed by bronze cast busts of all past presidents of the church. These transitional spaces in the grand circulation hall, especially at the upper levels, contain niches for sitting, contemplating or engaging in conversation.

In another shift of scale and descending movement, the space flows from the hall into the auditorium. Nine large skylights bring light into the auditorium, enhancing the sense that the Conference Center is a place of worship. The stage area in the auditorium can be adapted in a variety of configurations that accommodate the space's diverse purposes. The auditorium, while vast, is intimate, simultaneously being comfortable and impressive. The experience of attending a conference in the center auditorium is enhanced dramatically by feeling a part of a larger collective purpose, being one within in a congregation of 21,000-plus members of the church. This connection to a larger collective is reinforced by the geometry of the seating and the ceiling – a concaved oval cradling shape. The carefully designed, yellow-hued lighting system coupled with the deep red tones of pattern-matched cherry wood paneling comprising the walls and trim reinforces the warmth of the space. The auditorium is the nucleus of the building, but only in so far as its purpose is to connect the message within to the world without. As a place of broadcast, an understanding emerges while attending conferences that this architectural experience is just as much about being connected to other present attendees as it is about feeling part of a worldwide membership. With an international audience, the LDS Conference Center broadcasts to over eleven million members in eighty languages throughout the world who are watching and listening simultaneously.

Along with its various meetings and performances, the Conference Center is the new home of the world renowned Mormon Tabernacle Choir. The auditorium is the place where its hymns and anthems are sung, recorded and broadcast. Music for the faithful is of paramount importance; the state of the art, acoustically-enhanced auditorium is accented with a beautifully crafted 125-stacked-pipe organ. The quality and power of the sound that emanates from the choir and its accompanying organ is remarkable, unique and breathtaking.

At the conclusion of a session of conference, one ascends from the auditorium back to the grand circulation hall and out to the roof garden. In addition to enjoying the unique garden-like setting with varied vegetation, viewers can look to Temple Square below and then raise their eyes to the valley and the world beyond. The crescendo of the spatial sequence is the final journey down the exterior stairs: one literally cascades from level to level, finally reaching the entry plaza. The significance and excitement of this experience is magnified by the sheer volume of people descending in unison. While the

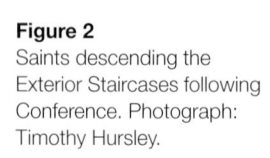

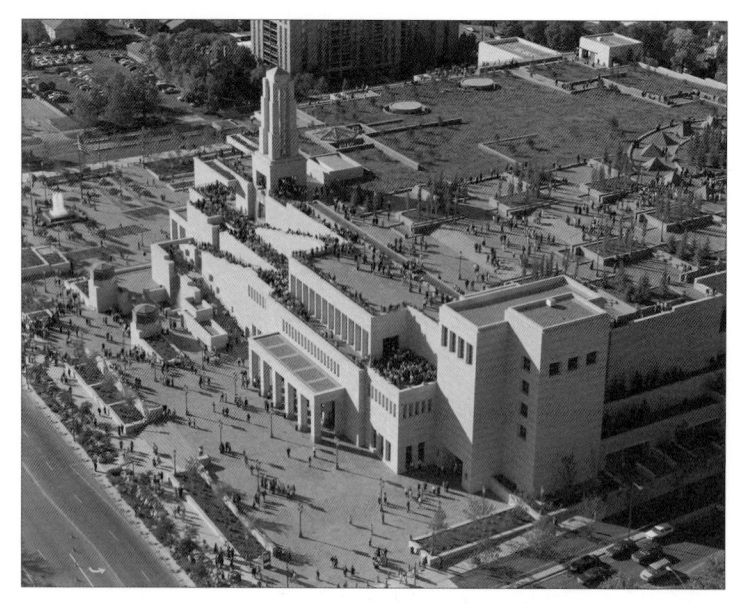

**Figure 2**
Saints descending the Exterior Staircases following Conference. Photograph: Timothy Hursley.

entry sequence to the center from the street plaza is somewhat alienating, the experience of descent after a unifying spiritual session of prophetic speeches and music is inclusive, exciting, communal and purpose filled.

## Joint Conclusion

In many ways the Conference Center is a building struggling with precedents. Regardless of its referential architectural language, the Center for the members of the Church of Jesus Christ of Latter-day Saints is a building of meaning, connecting its leaders, music and religious culture with its membership worldwide. It is a building that is deeply rooted to its locale and, simultaneously, global in perspective. In that respect it is a building that is without precedent.

## Notes

1. The senior design architect for the church was Leland Gray. The Portland, Oregon-based Zimmer Gunsul Frasca Partnership assisted as design architect and Auerbach & Associates of San Francisco was responsible for theater design and architectural lighting. The conference center was completed in 2000.
2. Hinckley, Gordon B. Conference Center Dedicatory Prayer, October 2000.

# BOOK REVIEWS

# Cross-talk between the Senses

## David Howes

*The Handbook of Multisensory Processes*, edited by Gemma Calvert, Charles Spence and Barry E. Stein, Cambridge, MA: The MIT Press, 2004, 915 pages. HB 0-262-03321-6. $125.00.

*Visual Music: Synaesthesia in Art and Music Since 1900*, with contributions by Kerry Brougher, Olivia Mattis, Jeremy Strick, Ari Wiseman and Judith Zilzcer, London: Thames & Hudson, 2005, 272 pages, with 376 illustrations, 344 in color. HB 0-500-51217-5. £32.00.

David Howes is the author of *Sensual Relations: Engaging the Senses in Culture and Social Theory* (2003). He is Professor of Anthropology at Concordia University, Montreal, and Director of the Concordia Sensoria Research Team (http://alcor.concordia.ca/~senses), as well as a contributing editor to *The Senses and Society*. david.howes@sympatico.ca

It is commonly assumed that each sense has its proper sphere (e.g. sight is concerned with color, hearing with sound and taste with flavor). This modular conception of the sensorium is reflected in the analytic orientation of most current research in the psychology of perception with its "sense-by-sense" – or, one sensory modality at a time – approach to the study of perceptual processes. In recent years, however, a more interactive, relational approach to the understanding of how the senses function has begun to take shape as a result of the growing body of evidence that points to the "multisensory organization" or "integration" of the brain. As Calvert, Spence and Stein write in their introduction to *The Handbook of Multisensory Processes*,

> even those experiences that at first may appear to be modality-specific are most likely to have been influenced by activity in other sensory modalities, despite our lack of awareness of such interactions … [To] fully appreciate the processes underlying much of sensory perception, we must understand not only how information from each sensory modality is transduced and decoded along the pathways primarily devoted to that sense, but also how this information is modulated by what is going on in the other sensory pathways. (2004: xi-xii)

Examples of such modulation include the well-documented fact that, in noisy surroundings, speakers can be understood more easily if they can be seen as well as heard. This finding is readily explicable in terms of the redundancy hypothesis of classic information theory. However, the new multisensory psychology of perception probes deeper to explore the *relationships* among the component parts of a multisensory signal. For example, in the case of animal and human communication, redundant multisensory signals can be subclassified into those that produce responses in the receiver equivalent to the response to each unisensory component (*equivalence*) and those for which the response is superadditive – that is, which exceeds the response to the unisensory components (*enhancement*). Multisensory signals may also be made up of stimuli which convey different (i.e. nonredundant) information, as in the case of the McGurk effect, where seen lip-movements can alter which phoneme is heard for a particular sound (e.g., a sound of /ba/ tends to be perceived as /da/ when it is coupled with a visual lip movement associated with /ga/). In this instance, the response to the multisensory signal is new, qualitatively different from the response to either of the unisensory components, and thus demonstrates *emergence*. The relationship between the components of a multisensory signal may otherwise be one of *dominance* as in the ventriloquism effect (where the seen lip-movements of the dummy alter or "capture" the apparent location of the speech sounds) or *concatenation* (my term) as in the case of the reproductive behavior of male oriental fruit moths: such moths "need the visual presence of the female in combination with her pheromones before they will perform their most intricate courtship displays, and they need an additional tactile stimulus of a touch on the abdomen before they will copulate" (p. 235).

Many of the chapters in the *Handbook* use modern neuroimaging techniques to reveal the multiple sites of multisensory processing in the brain, including many regions long thought to be modality-specific or "primary sensory" areas (as distinct from the so-called higher order "associative areas" traditionally assumed to be responsible for the formation of unified percepts out of the diversity of inputs). In addition to demonstrating the functional interdependence of the modalities, a number of chapters point to their functional equivalence. For example, it is now clear that sensory-specific areas can be "recruited" or "remapped" by other sensory-specific areas in situations of sensory deprivation or intensive perceptual training. Thus, the visual cortex in blind individuals has been found to show activation in auditory tasks while the auditory cortex in deaf individuals can be activated by visual tasks.

> Of note, the quality of sensation associated with activating the visual cortex in congenitally blind individuals, or the auditory cortex in congenitally deaf individuals, appears to derive from the nature of inputs. That is, visual inputs are perceived as visual even when auditory cortex is activated [in the case of the blind, while the reverse holds true in the case of the deaf]... Furthermore, even in normal, nondeprived humans, there is evidence for extensive multisensory interactions whereby primary sensory areas of the cortex can be activated in a task-specific manner by stimuli of other modalities... Common to these findings is the principle that inputs recruit pathways, cortical areas, and networks within and between areas that process the information, and the sensoriperceptual modality associated with the input is driven by the nature of the input rather than by the cortical area activated per se. (p. 690)

Such evidence of adaptive processing, or "cross-modal plasticity," underscores the importance of adopting a relational approach to the study of the sensorium in place of assuming that the senses are structurally and functionally distinct.

Other chapters explore such issues as whether the sensory integration involved in speech perception is fundamentally the same or different from other kinds of multisensory integration (the same); whether the senses are differentiated at birth and become coordinated through experience – the developmental integration hypothesis – or are relatively unified at birth and become differentiated through development – the developmental differentiation hypothesis (neither – the formation of percepts in early development involves the "joint action of developmental integration and differentiation processes" (p. 658)); and whether the phenomenon of synesthesia (i.e. the union or crossing of the senses, e.g. hearing colors, tasting shapes) might not provide a better model for conceptualizing perceptual processes than the conventional sense-by-sense approach that has dominated research on the senses and sensations to date.

The condition of synesthesia is typically understood to be quite rare. The most commonly documented form, color-grapheme synesthesia (in which written words or letters are perceived as having particular colors) occurs in one in 2,000 people. To limit synesthesia to a congenital condition, however, would be myopic.[1] Synesthetic connections can be learned. Take the case of odor-taste synesthesia which, perhaps because it is such a common effect, has failed to attract much popular attention or scientific documentation. Yet the evidence is clear:

> the majority of people appear to experience odor-taste synaesthesia. First, *sweet* is one of the most common descriptors applied to odors… [Furthermore,] when smelling an odor, most people can more easily recognize a taste-like quality such as sweetness than more specific qualities such as strawberry- or banana-likeness. (p. 69)

When we speak of the odor of vanilla or strawberry as sweet are we speaking in metaphor rather than reporting an actual olfactory sensation? Not according to Stevenson and Oakes:

> The central argument of [their] chapter is that, as a result of eating and drinking, patterns of retronasal odor stimulation co-occur with oral stimulation, notably of the taste receptors, so that a unitary percept is produced by a process of either within-event associative learning or by a simple encoding as one event. Eating sweet vanilla-flavor ice cream will ensure that the retronasal odor of vanilla becomes associated with sweetness; on some later occasion the smell of vanilla will seem sweet, even if no conscious recollecton of eating ice cream comes to mind. (p.81)

In the concluding chapter of the *Handbook*, V.S. Ramachandran et al. also reject what they call the "metaphor explanation" of synesthetic perception, and proffer a physiological explanation having to do with the "cross-activation of brain maps" in its place. Such cross-activation may come about by two different mechanisms:

> (1) cross-wiring between adjacent [brain] areas, either through an excess of anatomical connections or defective pruning, or (2) excess activity in back-projections between successive stages in the hierarchy (caused by defective pruning or by disinhibition). (p. 872)

In the case of color-grapheme synesthesia – their chosen example – the brain areas corresponding to graphemes and colors are right next to each other in the fusiform gyrus, and the potential for excess cross-activation or "hyperconnectivity" as a result of some genetic mutation in those individuals who naturally experience this effect is therefore strongly indicated. Ramachandran et al. conclude that far from being a mere curiousity, synaesthesia deserves to be brought into mainstream neuroscience and cognitive psychology. Indeed, [precisely because the neural basis of synaesthesia is beginning to be understood – unlike in the case of metaphor] it may provide a crucial insight into some of the most elusive questions about the mind, such as the neural substrate (and evolution) of metaphor, language and thought itself. (p. 881)

There is much to be said for Ramachandran et al.'s "bottom-up" approach to the study of synesthesia, but I do not think the "top-down" approach, which would descend from the cultural (via the metaphorical) to the psychological to the physiological level of brain organization, should be dismissed out of hand. (In point of fact, owing to the selective focus of their academic discipline, neuropsychology, Ramachandran et al. never ascend through what they call "the hierarchy" as far as the cultural level.)[2] If we are to comprehend fully all this evidence of cross-talk between the senses, there needs to be more cross-talk between the disciplines, by which I mean the insights of anthropology and history into the *cultural mediation of sensation* must also form part of the conversation. As cultural psychiatrist Laurence Kirmayer observes concerning the hierarchical systems view of neural organization,

> contemporary cognitive neuroscience understands mind and experience as phenomena that emerge from neural networks at a certain level of complexity and organization. There is increasing recognition that this organization is not confined to the brain but also includes loops through the body and the environment, most crucially, through a social world that is culturally constructed. On this view, "mind" is located not in the brain but in the relationship of brain and body to the world (Kirmayer, forthcoming).

Ideally, Kirmayer goes on to state, "we want to be able to trace the causal links up and down this hierarchy in a seamless way," but for this to come about neuropsychologists, historians and anthropologists will first have to overcome the selective focus of their respective disciplines and engage in more "joint action" research, as it were.

Imagine what a "Cross-Cultural Handbook of Multisensory Processes" would look like. Instead of presuming sensory processes to be confined to the brain, it would start with the investigation of the culturally patterned "loops" through the environment – that is, with the *cultural modulation of perception*. A "top-down" or culturally sensitive approach to, say, synesthetic perception would begin by providing an inventory of the cultural practices and technologies that generate different sense ratios across different cultures and historical periods. For example, whether the incidence of color-grapheme synesthesia would be as high in an aural-oral society as it is in a visual-literate one, such as contemporary Western society is a good empirical question.[3] In the latter, words and letters are experienced as quiescent marks on paper or a computer screen, which renders them available for color-coding, whereas in the former words (being experienced aurally) might not tend to be seen so readily as they would be felt or smelled as well as heard. In my own ethnographic research in Papua New Guinea, I found evidence of audio-olfactory synesthesia. In many Melanesian languages one speaks of "hearing an aroma" (and this association is carried over in Pidgin English: "mi harim smel"). The reason for this could be that most communication takes place face-to-face (i.e. within olfactory range of the other) and odoriferous substances (e.g. the oil with which the body is anointed or chewed ginger) are used to augment the power of a person's presence and words. This finding counters Stevenson and Boakes' claim that "odors display taste properties but do not elicit auditory or visual sensations" (p. 73). This claim is also countered by the evidence for a form of color-odor synesthesia reported by Diana Young among the Anangu of Australia's Western Desert (see Young 2005).

Starting with examples such as these, which, I would note, are *practical* (i.e. supported by cultural practices that form part of the "loop" through which all sensations must pass) as well as metaphorical, neuropsychologists could well be inspired to discover all sorts of heretofore unsuspected cross-linkages between the senses wherever they may be localized in the brain.[4] This is a heady prospect, but it can only come about as a result of more cross-talk between the disciplines leading to the establishment of *cultural* neuropsychology as a recognized field of study. It bears noting that the same shift from a unisensory to a multisensory approach to the study of perception that pervades the *Handbook* has been sweeping the humanities and social sciences in recent years (as observed in "Introducing Sensory Studies" – the lead essay in the inaugural issue of *The Senses and Society*). This convergence or fusion of horizons gives me great hopes for the conversation envisioned here. Furthermore, while I must confess to often feeling out of my depth reading *The Handbook of Multisensory Processes*, I never ceased to marvel at the ingenuity of the experiments, or to admire the meticulousness of the reasoning involved in the interpretation of results in any of its fifty-four chapters. I would therefore recommend the *Handbook* as essential reading for any scholar interested in exploring the varieties of sensory experience in history and across cultures on account of the multiple models and questions it suggests for further archival or ethnographic research.[5]

*Visual Music: Synaesthesia in Art and Music Since 1900* is a beautifully illustrated catalog that accompanied the exhibition by the same name at The Museum of Contemporary Art, Los Angeles and the Hirshorn Museum and Sculpture Garden of the Smithsonian Institution in Washington in 2005. This groundbreaking study begins by presenting an "alternative history" of the abstract art of the past century by disclosing its debt to music. Because of the selective (visual) focus of conventional art history, the development of abstraction is commonly told in terms of avant-garde artists seeking to produce a non-representational – or "pure" – art that would be "freed from imitative constraints," without it being appreciated how much that movement was inspired and dependent in its formative stages on emulating the formal abstract structures of musical composition. Music had long been considered the most spiritually exalting and purest form of art on account of its ethereality, nonobjectivity and emotivity (or direct appeal to the affects), and it was the idea of visual art aspiring to "the condition of music" – that is, of creating "music for the eyes" – that inspired many of the pioneers of abstraction on both sides of the Atlantic, from Wassily Kandinsky and Paul Klee in Europe to Arthur Dove and Georgia O'Keefe in America. The rhythmic interplay of geometry and color in Kandinsky's later paintings (e.g. *Fuga (Fugue)*, 1914), and the synesthetic theory of painting he elaborated in *On the Spiritual in Art*, led one fellow artist to write "Kandinsky is attempting to paint the color of sound" (p. 35). Klee, for his part, transformed polyphony into abstract pictorial form (e.g. *Static-Dynamic Gradation*, 1923), while O'Keefe records that the impetus behind her organic abstractions (e.g. *Blue and Green Music*, 1921) came from attending an art class where students were required to draw while listening to music: "This gave me an idea that I was very interested to follow later – the idea that music could be translated into something for the eye" (p. 59).

The dream of the "unification of the arts" through "sensual compounding" which inspired these experiments in abstraction simultaneously exposed a major shortcoming intrinsic to the medium of painting: its immobility or static character. Musical compositions, of course, unfold through time. "Abstract film developed as if in direct response to this shortcoming," the authors claim (p. 19). The originators of abstract cinema, working in black and white, "elaborated sequences of geometric forms that moved across the screen and through time, as would a sequence of sounds," and then, as technologies of color film and soundtracks developed, their successors, such as Oskar Fischinger, were able to bring

> color, form, and sound together to create extended compositions that bore occasional resemblance to the work of the earlier generations of abstract painters while taking full advantage of the crucial element of time and incorporating sound and music to create a fully synaesthetic experience. (p. 19)

The most famous example of this genre is, of course, the Disney Studio animated motion picture *Fantasia* (1940), in which Fischinger had a hand. In addition to propelling the synchronization of the senses to new heights, *Fantasia* signaled a fundamental change in the direction of visual music: the change "from an avant-garde practice toward a modern mass-cultural phenomenon" (p. 111).

The changeover in visual music from avant-garde practice to pop culture continued apace in the 1950s and 1960s with the phenomenon of the light show (e.g. the Vortex concerts), which drew together a wide variety of practices – from performance art to scientific experiments, from coffeehouse jazz concerts to psychedelic drugs – to create

> an immersive visual and sound experience. The light show offered a neutral place in which high art and popular culture, abstraction and representation, the scientific and the spiritual, the electronic and natural, and the visual and aural could all be collaged together in a vast swirling eddy of overlapping sensations. It was the ultimate synaesthetic experience, one that attempted through the hallucinogenic to blur the distinction between sound and image, interior and exterior. (p. 159)

In their effort to trace the "successive unfolding" of the idea of visual music – from abstraction, to abstraction in motion, to total immersion – the contributors to the catalog also canvas many other artistic expressions and inventions besides those surveyed above, such as the color organ, optical printer, contemporary installation art and digital media, as well as diverse controversies (e.g. over the validity of the analogy between specific colors and specific musical notes or keys in the first place). The catalog is also crowned with a brilliant chapter on color music from a musical perspective, which reverses the drift of all the other chapters, and a very informative "Chronology" that, by documenting the successive engagements with and elaborations of the notion of visual music on both sides of the Atlantic (and from coast to coast in the United States), gives substance to the claim that this stylistic strain, while

> not the single mode through which music and the visual arts have interacted over the past century ... is certainly the most consistent ... continuing to find new arenas for aesthetic exploration even as other, more famous movements and styles [e.g. Cubism through Abstract Expressionism] eventually faltered. Its longevity can be explained above all by the fact that it required technology for its fulfillment. (p. 18)

While I am in deep sympathy with the first branch of this argument, I must register my dissent from the progressivist conclusion in the second branch to the effect that the promise of synesthesia

– the compounding of the senses leading to spiritual awakening as imagined by Kandinsky – was "fulfilled" by technology – that is, by the synchronization of the senses in film and other so-called multi-media. For such media foregrounded certain sensory ratios – most notably the audio-visual – while screening out others and thus limited "mind" or consciousness in the very act of extending or projecting it outwards. The tradition of visual music could equally well be interpreted as involving a contraction of the synesthetic paradigm.[6] There exist other sensory ratios than those hypostasized in the technological dynamo of our audio-visual civilization. At the same time, *Visual Music* does prove that the history of art (or of music) is best practiced with two senses, rather than one – and thus agrees with the central theoretical and methodological claims of *The Handbook of Multisensory Processes*.

## Notes

1. The ethnomusicologist Steve Feld once remarked to me that limiting synesthesia to those who are congenitally susceptible to this effect would be like restricting music to those with perfect pitch. It cannot be so confined. But to qualify this assertion, and anticipate my discussion of Ramachandran's position in what follows, let me note that I concur with Ramachandran's view that synesthesia is sensory or perceptual, not conceptual or metaphorical. It is not just another trope. However, by ignoring the *practical* (i.e. culturally patterned and learned) dimensions of synesthesia, it seems to me that Ramachandran forecloses an important avenue of inquiry into the genesis of this effect at the level of the individual and its shaping or expression at the cultural level.
2. Ramachandran et al. are not alone. There is but one reference in the whole *Handbook* to cross-cultural variation in the modulation of perception: apparently, the McGurk effect is significantly weaker in Japanese than in American perceivers (p. 207).
3. Or even earlier periods of Western culture. For example, a form of audio-grapheme synesthesia has been described for the Renaissance: "In a person's handwriting, Erasmus claimed, he could hear that person's very voice" (Smith 2004: 21–41 at 28).
4. That is, proximity of brain areas would no longer be the determinative criterion (*pace* Ramachandran et al.) -- as indeed it is not, given all the evidence of cross-modal activation, feed forward and back-projection processes that has begun to emerge.
5. A number of sensorially-minded anthropologists have already opened this conversation with neuropsychology and made significant headway exploring "the question of how far back into the genesis of bodily experience [or activation of brain areas] cultural worlds can reach" (Kirmayer, forthcoming): most notably, Hinton and Hinton (2002), Young (2005), and Downey (2005).

6. Imagine how different the history of abstraction in art would have been had it started with Des Esseintes' "mouth organ" (a collection of liqueurs each analogous to a musical note, which the protagonist of Huysmans' *À rebours* played upon his palette) in place of the color organ. This example is cited in *Visual Music* but dismissed as too "literal" (p. 16). That audio-gustatory synesthesia can, in fact, form the basis of a highly abstract art is evidenced by the case of Indian aesthetics and cosmology (see Pinard 1991; Schechner 2001). For a good overview of the full range of sensory combinations explored by Western artists prior to the cinematic turn see *The Color of Angels* (Classen 1998).

**References**

Classen, Constance. 1998. *The Color of Angels: Cosmology, Gender and the Aesthetic Imagination*. London and New York: Routledge.

Downey, Greg. 2005. "Seeing with a 'Sideways Glance': Visuomotor Knowing and the Plasticity of Perception." Paper presented at the "Ways of Knowing" conference, St Andrew's University.

Hinton, Devon and Hinton, Susan. 2002. "Panic Disorder, Somatization, and the New Cross-Cultural Psychiatry: The Seven Bodies of a Medical Anthropology of Panic" *Culture, Medicine and Psychiatry* 26: 155–78.

Kirmayer, Laurence J. n.d. "On the Cultural Mediation of Pain." In S. Coakley and K. Shelemay (eds), *Pain and Its Transformations*. Cambridge, MA: Harvard University Press. Forthcoming.

Pinard, Sylvain. 1991. "A Taste of India: On the Role of Gustation in the Hindu Sensorium." In David Howes (ed.), *The Varieties of Sensory Experience*. Toronto: University of Toronto Press.

Schechner, Richard. 2001. "Rasaesthetics." *The Drama Review* 45(3): 27–50.

Smith, Bruce R. 2004. "Listening to the Wild Blue Yonder: The Challenges of Acoustic Ecology." In Veit Erlmann (ed.), *Hearing Cultures: Essays on Sound, Listening and Modernity*. Oxford: Berg.

Young, Diana. 2005. "The Smell of Greenness: Cultural Synaesthesia in the Western Desert." *Etnofoor* 18(1): 61–77.

# A Sense of Things to Come: On the Emergent Dialogue between Contemporary Art and Anthropology

**Andrew Irving**

*Contemporary Art and Anthropology*, by Arnd Schneider and Christopher Wright, eds., Oxford and New York: Berg, 2005, 320 pages. ISBN 1845201035. $34.95.

Andrew Irving is a lecturer in Visual Anthropology at Manchester University. His research explores how the world appears to people close to death, particularly in relation to the perception and aesthetic appreciation of time, existence and otherness.
irving2000@gmail.com

*Contemporary Art and Anthropology* brings together artists and anthropologists to consider current representational practices, and explores how the creative dialogues and interdisciplinary tensions that emerge when artists and anthropologists engage with one another's practices might shed new light upon sociocultural life and aesthetics. In their Introduction, Schneider and Wright set out "an agenda for future collaborations based upon examples of radical experiments from contemporary art and anthropology. Our main argument is that anthropology's iconophobia and self-imposed restriction of visual expression to text-based models needs to be overcome by a critical engagement with a range of material and sensual practices in the contemporary arts" (p. 4). Hence, they urge us to engage our senses through such things as "books" made of out of iron oxide and linseed oil that evoke the haptic and olfactory dimensions of reading, and "ethnopoetic" displays that highlight the aural rhythms and synaesthetic potential implied in visual text.

The senses are not the exclusive preserve of artists. By virtue of the nervous system, every human being is continually subjected to different sensory and aesthetic experiences. A central question posed by Schneider and Wright therefore concerns how to better represent and understand the multisensoriality of social life and experience. It is instructive here to recall the etymology of the word "aesthetics": the original meaning of *aisthitikos* was "perceptive by feeling," suggesting not art but reality – or rather a *corpo*reality, since it is through the faculties of taste, touch, hearing, seeing and smell that we come to know and understand the world. For Schneider and Wright this is "the challenge of practice" they hope to address through the chapters collected for this volume.

Victor Turner advocated using drama and performance to bring anthropology to life. In "Artists in the Field," George Marcus notes that Turner was particularly interested in how issues of mind and emotion could be evoked through the aesthetics of performance. Marcus recounts how he himself had abandoned hope that the aesthetic implications of the watershed volume *Writing Culture: The Politics and Poetics of Ethnography* (1996) would be developed by anthropologists, since its effect largely focused attention on issues of textual and ethnographic authority. In Turner's footsteps, Marcus' co-author, theater practitioner Fernando Calzadilla, attempts to realize anthropology's theoretical, aesthetic and sensory concerns in the field by creating a multisensorial structure in a Venezuelan marketplace consisting of pipes, plastic sheets, asphalt, onion sacks and carrier bags in collaboration with the market's workers. The aim being to emphasize the material affects and occasional violence of everyday market life under the looming presence of the Venezuelan oil industry.

In "The Ancient American Roots of Abstraction," Argentinean sculptor and painter Cesar Paternosto offers an alternative take on the South American landscape by mixing different earthy and sandy-grey pigments combined with marble powder to obtain subtle textural differences that speak equally to touch and vision. These textures register the lingering effects of Paternosto's being "in the field" – traveling around the Andean mountains and witnessing Incan monoliths, temples and sculptural forms.

Many contributors explore how art can be used to supplement and provide a richer understanding of the worlds represented in academic theories and models. Michael Richardson, for example, uses the work of Czech painter Josef Šíma to grapple seriously with the notion that reality is not simply constituted by independently observable material components and needs art to expose the immaterial dimensions of being, including dreams and the imaginary. Susanne Küchler explores the borders of vision and cognition which are revealed when mathematics and art are placed in dialogue. The knot-sculptures she examines are collaborative hybrids that cannot be comprehended within the confines of either discipline alone. Küchler then asks what might be gained by looking at art through the lens of mathematics and science and the intriguing implications this holds for visual anthropology.

Nicholas Thomas considers another kind of intersection, in which different artists are brought together to reveal the complex flows of culture, displacement and living history that are inscribed on the surfaces of the skin in tattoos. These flows are embodied in artistic encounters – for example between the skin and the camera, whereby Polynesian tattoos become an object of photographic interest and come to form a second skin that enters into the representative milieu. Thomas gives the example of contemporary Samoan artist Greg Semu's portraits of himself as an ironically displaced subject of a nineteenth-century ethnological photograph. A further "self-portrait of displacement" is provided in Elizabeth Edwards' discussion of Mohini Chandra's installations, photographs and video works, *Travels in a New World* and *Album Pacifica*. Chandra's point of departure is that of multiple displacements, starting with her family being uprooted from India and transported to Fiji by the British, and their subsequent diasporic movements around the globe. Edwards understands these works, and the journeys they represent, not simply as idiosyncratic and fragmentary articulations of issues of homeland, identity and belonging but in terms of a method and ethnography appropriate to understanding the contemporary world.

Jonathan Friedman's chapter concerns contemporary artist Carlos Capelán, whose works make reference to anthropology's diverse modes of appropriation and representation. Friedman expands the definition of appropriation to include the colonization of other people's "experiential" worlds, which he somewhat tendentiously claims is something that no "real" artist would do; however, what distinguishes the real from the counterfeit remains unexplored. The themes of misconstruction and misappropriation are further dealt with in Chris Pinney's illuminating chapter "Moon and Mother: Francesco Clemente's Orient" and Schneider's chapter on "Appropriations." Pinney highlights how contemporary Indian-influenced art often fails to engage with contemporary Indian realities by excluding the political and economic "frame" that surrounds the artwork. Thus appropriations of India posit a different and static temporality (based on romantic and Disneyfied tropes of Indian history, myth and alterity) insofar as recent social, political and revolutionary change within Indian culture rarely enters into the "picture," leading Pinney to call for a "re-orientation" of the orient. Schneider argues that the incorporation of cultural differences into material artifacts, such as in the encounter between Picasso and the "magic" of African sculpture, is not simply a defining characteristic of twentieth-century art, but also of *anthropology*. That anthropology appropriates material artifacts for museums is well known, but Schneider points out how anthropology, by way of an academic alchemy, turns myths, rituals, social life, persons and their kin relations into ethnographic, literary artifacts for wider academic consumption. Thus Pinney and Schneider raise the important question of what kinds of appropriation are appropriate for twenty-first century artists and anthropologists.

One way to avoid this dilemma is to appropriate oneself. In an essay on contemporary artist Susan Hiller, art critic Denise Robinson considers how people move from one condition of being to another, for example through altered states and phantasms. Hiller herself made this journey by transforming herself from a practicing anthropologist to a practicing artist in response to what she deemed anthropology's intellectual, economic and political colonization of other peoples. Art, she suggests, "with no overt political content can sensitise us politically" (p. 73), thereby offering a different and perhaps more ethically grounded way of interacting with and understanding other persons. A further reflective gaze is provided by a specially commissioned photographic essay by Dave Lewis, taking the Anthropology Department at the University of East London as its ethnographic site, and a dialogue between various protagonists of "fieldwork" and "tracking evidence" movements in the contemporary art of the last twenty years, including Rainer Wittenborn, Claus Biegert, Nikolaus Lang, and Rimer Cardillo.

*Contemporary Art and Anthropology* questions many traditional disciplinary presuppositions and figures as a radical manifesto that advocates a more sensorially-grounded and collaborative approach to cultural analysis and aesthetics. The combination of art and anthropology working together, and sometimes in tension, has the power to reveal aspects of sensory experience, social life and material culture that would otherwise remain hidden. However, this collaboration must take place not merely at the level of theory and representation but also fieldwork method and practice. For while anthropology might be considered a "fieldwork science/documentary art," after reading this volume we can see how anthropology might more ambitiously be transformed into a "fieldwork art/documentary art" dedicated to expressing the sensory dimensions of thinking and being. Such a move recalls the approach of Victor Turner, whose own attempts to combine ritual, performance and ethnography anticipate many of the concerns raised throughout this volume.

The book provocatively questions established notions of what constitutes "anthropological" as well as "artistic" knowledge. If different sensory experiences embody and facilitate different kinds of knowledge, then we need to develop new methods and more sensually appropriate forms of representation that are not simply based on the correspondence theory of truth, which restricts the empirical to the visible. It is in its practical and methodological implications that the book excels and distinguishes itself from the existing anthropological canon on art, while simultaneously offering a much-needed alternative fieldwork research methods manual to counteract conventional social scientific research methods that privilege certain ways of knowing and rarely account for the bodily and sensory dimensions of social life.

Not that the book succeeds on all counts. Indeed, artists have long known that failure is essential to the creative process. Perhaps anthropologists also need to embrace failure as being fundamental to both fieldwork and writing. For example, instead of lamenting the impossibility of representing and translating the multisensuality of social life, fieldwork experience and material culture by way of language, this alleged aporia could better be explored as a creative tension that generates new and multiple forms of thinking and writing about our embodied and sensory experiences of the world rather than being an obstacle to a single "truth." Different senses reveal different truths and the co-presence of different sensory modalities within life and art; alongside their refusal to be translated into linear text, allows us to grasp the complexity of our object of study in new ways. It is by refusing to accord a foundational status of truth to any particular sense or mode of representation that a greater and more rounded "sense" of the world emerges.

While commenting extensively on the relationship between contemporary art and anthropology the book fails to fully problematize its central subject – that of the contemporaneous *vis-à-vis* art, material culture and aesthetic affects. For anthropologists are rightly wary of the inherent temporalization of cultural difference whereby non-western practices, artistic or otherwise, are seen as some throwback to earlier, more earthy, more sensual, more primitive forms of humanity. Whenever temporalizations of difference, processes of categorization and restrictions of the interpretative multiplicity of art occur we have to look at the power operating behind the scenes, which here is the western art world/industry, whose terms anthropologists cannot accept uncritically.

These criticisms aside, *Contemporary Art and Anthropology* is an excellent commentary on current representational practices *and* possibilities. For those interested in the senses the book is good to "think with" and offers a rich and varied attempt to *use* rather than merely study art, in order to explore, evoke, provoke and better understand the fluidity, complexity and depth of social life; moreover it offers a plethora of essential new perspectives for the study and practice of art, aesthetics and anthropology. It is to an artist, Jean Genet, as quoted by Denise Robinson, that the last words should be left: "Art should exalt only those truths which are not demonstrable, and which are even false, those which we cannot carry to their ultimate conclusions without absurdity, without negating both them and yourself. They will never have the good or bad fortune to be applied" (p. 73).

# EXHIBITION AND CONFERENCE REVIEWS

# Even-handedness

The Prisoners' Inventions
I Space Gallery, Chicago, Illinois

**Kevin Henry**

**Kevin Henry is coordinator of the product design program at Columbia College Chicago. A practicing industrial designer, writer and curator his interests revolve around the overlaps of design, studio art practice and the social sciences. Current theoretical research focuses on the relationships of language evolution to that of artifacts.
khenry@colum.edu.**

"Prisoners' Inventions" is an exhibition that manages to deliver a level of naturalism similar to that of a great documentary film while engaging the viewer in an immersive interactive experience. The work is a collaboration between the Chicago collective Temporary Services and the pseudonymous inmate Angelo. The artists have recreated a range of prison artifacts (as well as a prison cell) based on rough schematic drawings and annotations provided by Angelo – an act that serves simultaneously to separate the original artifacts from the larger context of prison life while drawing them closer to the world of designed and manufactured objects. Standing in that tiny cell (door wide open) quickly convinced me that sensory deprivation is the flip side of pain in terms of its effect on consciousness – whereas pain succeeds through relentless presence, deprivation succeeds through relentless absence, and deprivation is clearly at the heart of incarceration. For the prisoners in this exhibition the least intrusive act of defiance (but perhaps the most subversive) is to "create" with their own hands the artifacts denied them from the "outside" world. This drive to creatively utilize that part of

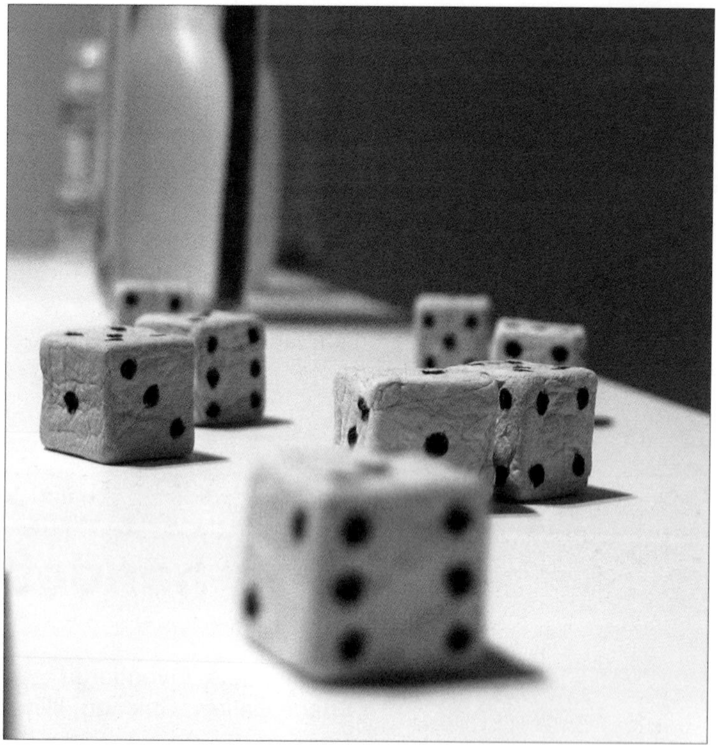

Exhibition Review

**Figure 1**
Toilet paper dice.
Photograph by Kevin Henry

their body so strongly connected in the popular consciousness with criminality lifts these otherwise mundane objects to another level while the manner in which the objects are created and the inventive use of material adds poignancy and intrigue. Henri Focillon's book *In Praise of Hands* sums it up very nicely: "In the artist's studio are to be found the hand's trials, experiments, and divinations, the age-old memories of the human race, which has not forgotten the privilege of working with the hands." In "The Prisoners' Inventions," the hand, that pre-linguistic communicator and form-giver (so often portrayed as shackled, cuffed or tied when associated with prison), becomes the silent center of the exhibition.

While Angelo has not invented all the objects he has served as the primary conduit in visualizing them. The net result is a rich, almost anthropological recording of prison life and the archetypical artifacts commonly found within prisons throughout the USA and, by inference, in any penal setting. The act of encoding the inventions in paper drawings (the only medium of communication available to Angelo) so that they may later be realized in the 'free context' of the gallery adds another layer, requiring a conceptual shift on the part of the viewer. It is easy to ask what these artifacts have to do with art or why they are presented in this context. The answer is harder to find, and therein lies part of the show's broader impact.

The work assumes an almost monastic quality in its simplicity and lack of ornament – much like a group of nineteenth-century tools from a Shaker village or artifacts exhumed and placed under vitrines in a natural history museum. The objects manage to celebrate the quotidian aspects of prison life while contextualizing our own long history of tool making. I often found myself marveling at the ingenuity of material usage without thinking much about the realities of prison life: the deprivation or the danger. As in many museum exhibitions, there was a muteness to the objects that belied their current everyday use in prisons across the country. These are not artifacts whose purpose has been lost to history but rather contemporary objects and tools cobbled together from readily available materials to satisfy a range of timeless needs.

While the word "invention" generally invokes new technology or creation, in this setting, the focus is really on re-invention. This is also part of the lure of the exhibition: as humans we are naturally drawn to the challenge of making do with available materials to recreate the typical artifacts we have come to rely on for survival or just as plain old creature comforts to increase our quality of life. We can see it daily in any catastrophe or disaster film or in the recent spate of Reality TV shows. Such an encounter can lull us out of our consumerist slumber to witness firsthand real individuals using their wits to solve simple problems that no longer register with us or to create common artifacts whose origins or even reasons for existing may elude us.

The artifacts serve the additional purpose of inventorying the important things in a prison while allowing the viewer the opportunity to provide any number of possible narratives to connect them all. Part of this connection is, no doubt, the ingenuity with which deprivation is transcended, but another part clearly unites the viewer with the human desire to be creative regardless of the situation. This is not an exhibition preaching a message of prison reform or hidden social agendas as much as one focused on revealing the humanity in us all regardless of our context.

The work ranges from the sacred to the profane or the mundane. Accompanying Angelo's drawings are often texts that provide additional details of prison life as well as descriptions of how various objects are constructed or materials obtained. These accounts quickly reveal the fact that here, inside the impenetrable walls of a prison, we find, oddly enough, a village. One of the inmates is skilled in working with string to make the best wicks while another jury-rigs electronics and still another works wonders with tape of all sorts. What happens outside the prison walls is quickly replicated inside. We begin to see a microcosmology reflecting the larger 'free' macro organism beyond the walls and razor wire. The main difference (and this is truly a big difference) is that time is no longer counted as money. This is a smaller universe reflective of medieval values nestled inside a larger capitalist universe.

Exhibition Review

**Figure 2**
Toilet paper chess set.
Photograph by Kevin Henry.

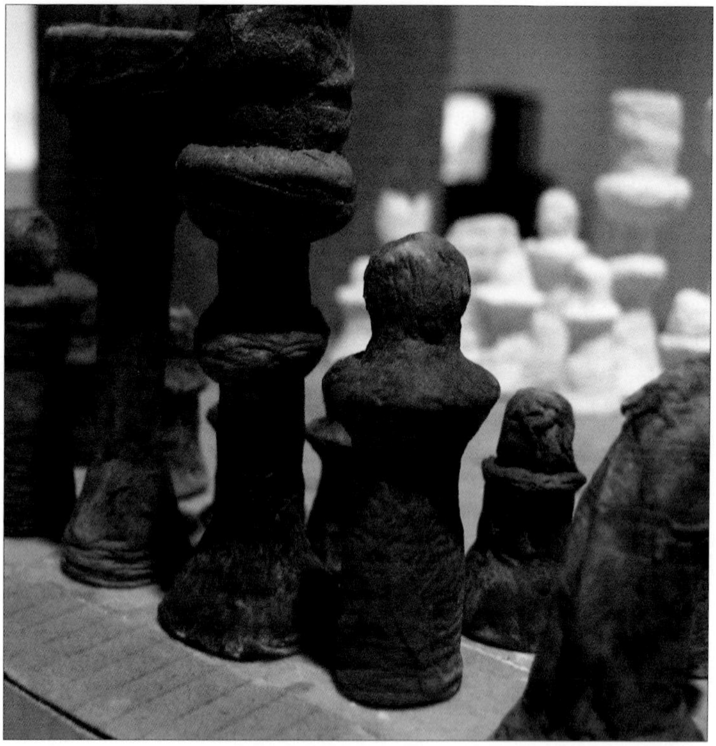

The most profound aspect of the show is the magic of some of the inventions. Like any small island ecology, the prison has certain raw material in excess while other materials are extremely hard to come by. Toilet paper is to the prison ecology what wood is to the forest ecology, and is therefore one of the most commonly 'found' resources. As a result many of the objects are created with it, from simple containers fashioned out of wadded toilet paper and clear tape to the most elegant object in the show – a toilet paper chess set. The real beauty of the chess pieces, however, comes through the ironic softening of the war metaphor (implicit in chess) once it is reinvented in paper. The only resemblance to a normal chess set is the iconic typology of the pieces. The aggressive thud of wood, metal, onyx, pewter or hard plastic on the game board as a psychological tactic against one's opponent has forever been removed. Not only has the game been rendered silent (by necessity no doubt) but also gentler, adding an almost Zen-like aura to it.

Dice have gone through a similar regeneration, removing that most fundamental of sounds – tumbling. Gone is the thrill the sound alone invokes as the dice careen against cardboard or wooden game boards before slowly stopping to reveal their values. These paper dice certainly roll (having the same six sides) but as though in a silent film. In fact many of the prisoners' inventions, whether by necessity or subterfuge, operate in a world that is silent – yet another reminder of the repressive nature of prisons and the determined human will to subvert or at least temporarily rise above that repression. Temporary Services, for their part, have reinforced this aura of silence through the many videos they have lovingly created of the actual fabrication of several of the pieces in the exhibition that are displayed on several monitors set around the gallery. Shot in a matter-of-fact method with a simple neutral background and tightly focused on an anonymous set of hands shaping the artifacts, much like an industrial film, the videos bring a level of naturalism seen in films like Robert Bresson's *A Man Escaped* or Chantal Akerman's *Jeanne Dielman, 23 Quai du Commerce, 1080 Bruxelles*.

The videos work as both Do-It-Yourself instruction sets and documentary pieces proving the origins and methods of the work in the exhibition to be true to life. These videos are an eerie reminder of the reality of prison: its anonymity and sensual deprivation. The video demonstrating the manufacture of the dice is especially poignant: silent hands tightly focused within the camera frame repeatedly mold the paper softened in a mix of sugar water to achieve the final form of each die – a task much like that of a pastry chef molding a petit four or some other delicate pastry.

The full effect of the exhibition, including the artifacts, the process videos and the replicated prison cell (approximate both in terms of footprint and actual materials), is simultaneously claustrophobic and expansive. While the gallery provides a space for the activities and artifacts to spill out of the small cell, adding both breathing room and natural light to view the artifacts, they remain compacted on their pedestals, full of the energy of clandestine creation and use. The show succeeds at providing a strangely voyeuristic perspective onto another reality while reflecting our common humanity – half window, half mirror. Finally the creation/consumption mode implicit in the artifacts serves to remind the viewer of that most critical of human needs: our sensual ritualistic need to engage in making and consuming our own handiwork.

# Celebrate the 10th anniversary of
# Fashion Theory

## The Journal of Dress, Body & Culture

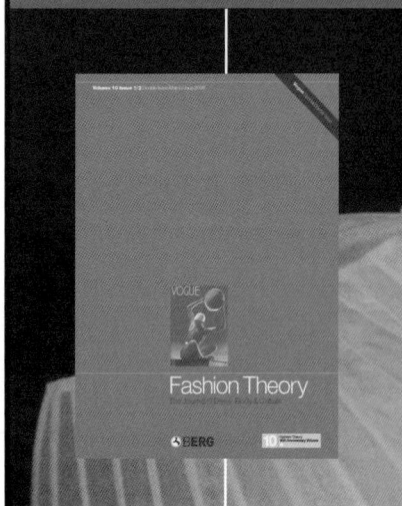

**Edited by Dr. Valerie Steele,** Director of the Museum at the Fashion Institute of Technology in New York

'A fine addition to academic institutions with cultural studies programs; essential for those with special collections in fashion and costume.' **Library Journal**

'Fashion Theory is both chic and serious –yes, and sexy, too.' **Times Higher Education Supplement**

'For those who dismiss fashion as frivolous, here's proof otherwise.' **Harper's Bazaar**

Reprinted courtesy of Arkadius

Since its launch in 1997 as the first journal devoted to the intellectual understanding of the dressed body, *Fashion Theory* has remained at the vanguard of international fashion scholarship.

**Celebrate Fashion Theory's 10th anniversary with**
- NEW online only pricing - $200 / £115
- Volumes 1-6 will be available online from March 2007, completing the online archive
- A NEW annotated index of all articles in Volume 10 Issue 4!
- A NEW *Fashion Theory* Reader in 2007 – selected highlights from 10 years!
- A NEW *Fashion Theory* Set – 27 issues for 15% off! ONLY $665 / £375!

**Indexed by:**
IBSS, DAAI, ART Bibliographies Modern, H.W. Wilson Art Index, AIO, Sociological Abstracts, ISI Web of Science/Arts & Humanities Citation Index, THOMSON ISI Current Contents Connect/Arts & Humanities, MLA Bibliography.

Published 4 times a year in March, June, September and December.

| FASHION THEORY | |
| --- | --- |
| ISSN 1362-704X | 1 year |
| Individual Subscription | |
| Print only, does not include online access. | £46 / $79 |
| Institutional Print and Online | |
| Includes online access Vol. 7-10. | £140 / $250 |
| Online only | |
| Includes online access Vol. 7-10. | £115+VAT / $200 |
| The Print Set | |
| Volumes 1-7 | £375 / $665 |

**BERG**

Order online at www.bergpublishers.com or call +44(0)1767 604951
Institutional subscriptions include online access through www.IngentaConnect.com
To order a sample copy please contact enquiry@bergpublishers.com
View issue 7.1 free online at www.ingentaconnect.com

# Synesthesia Soirées

Four Soirées around the theme of Synaesthesia. Convened by Pieter Verstraete and Maaike Bleeker, Amsterdam School for Cultural Analysis (ASCA), Amsterdam, February–March, 2006.

## Maaike Bleeker

Maaike Bleeker is an assistant professor in theater studies, University of Amsterdam and an NWO (Netherlands Organisation for Scientific Research) research fellow (project titled: *See Me, Feel Me, Think Me: The Body of Semiotics*). For the past ten years she has worked as a dramaturge with various directors, choreographers and visual artists.
m.a.bleeker@uva.nl

Pieter Verstraete is preparing a Ph.D.-thesis within the Ph.D.-program of the Amsterdam School for Cultural Analysis (ASCA). His project is (provisionally) titled "The Frequency of Imagination: a Perceptual-Narrative Study of the Relations between Sound, Performance Text and Theatrical Space."
p.m.g.verstraete@uva.nl

The principle of synesthesia describes the correspondence of different sense perceptions, their interconnectedness, the possibility of transference, conversion and translation of one sense into others or the synthesis of separate experiences. In literature, synesthesia commonly denotes a metaphorical expression of the multisensory nature of experiences like those described by Baudelaire: "It is not only in dreams, or in the mild delirium which precedes sleep, but it is even awakened when I hear music – that perception of an analogy and an intimate connection between colours, sounds and perfumes" (Shaw-Miller 2002: 55). In neurobiology, synesthesia is explained as a perceptual anomaly, as in the case of a woman who experiences shapes accompanying smells, such that the smell of wintergreen evokes "ragged edges," and peanut butter smells like "things falling down and backward" (Harrison 2001). As an artistic project, synesthesia played an important part in the late nineteenth and early twentieth centuries, when it inspired many artists who aimed at involving all the senses in a synesthetic totality (e.g. Wagner's *Gesamtkunstwerk*), or at addressing one sensory channel through another (e.g. Kandinsky's attempts at evoking sound through color). This historical project went through a highly experimental phase in the 1920s and 1930s with the films of Oskar Fischinger, John and James Whitney and Thomas Wilfred. Its heyday appeared to come to an end in the 1960s in the wake of psychedelic light shows and synesthetic concerts with audiovisual synthesizers that made the participant's physical presence and experience the key to synesthesia. Many of these artistic projects were motivated by a holistic believe in a higher cosmic unity, the desire for a closer touch at reality, or the belief in the possibility of a mystical-religious transformation through an experience that transcends everyday sense perception.

Although seemingly "outdated" now, these experiments influenced immersive installation art as we know it today. Moreover, these synesthetic experiments question the rather complex nature and ambiguous relationships between the senses. New scientific insights, both theoretical and experimental, into the inevitable impurity of sensory perception and the interconnectedness of what we often experience as separate faculties, point to the need to reconsider the function and operations of synesthesia. Rather than a mind anomaly or mystical experience, it seems that synesthesia is the norm of every sense perception, of imagination and creativity. We read novels visually, experience music through muscular sensuality and palpate paintings with our eyes.

These observations formed the starting point for four soirées around the theme of synesthesia organized by Pieter Verstraete and myself as part of the research program of the Amsterdam School for Cultural Analysis (ASCA) at the University of Amsterdam (February 20 and 27, March 6 and 13, 2006). Instead of conceiving of synesthesia merely as a metaphorical use of the senses (as it is commonly treated in literature), we proposed to push the concept and its applicability to different fields of cultural analysis by re-assessing it

- as a tool for addressing multiple senses, wired with each other in still unexplored ways (related to issues of the sensorium, anthropology of the senses, a trans/metasensorial model)
- as a way of understanding the fading boundaries between the material and the immaterial world (like instances of haptic, tactile or corporeal experiences, imagination, immersion, virtuality and artistic creativity)
- as an exploration of different media (intermediality) via different disciplines (interdisciplinarity)
- as a challenge to the traditional status of the (visual/acoustic) image, available for discursive thought as content of knowledge
- as a catalyst for related methodological questions (such as synthesis v. analysis, embodied knowledge, practice as research, performative narratology).

Each evening, three or four scholars presented case studies attached to a different theoretical aspect of the over-arching theme posed above. Each presenter proposed one text for inclusion in the reader we prepared for the soirées, to be read in advance by the participants. The presentations were followed by dinner and extensive discussions. Each evening was organized around a specific theme. The first soirée was entitled *Sound and Vision*. Presenters included: John Neubauer, "Romantic Synaesthesia," Chris Balme, "Seeing Sound," Carolyn Birdsall, "Gesamtkunstwerk as Total World of Hearing" and, Marga van Mechelen, "The Battle of the DJ and the VJ, or of Sound and Image." The second soirée was entitled *Intersensory Experience*, with presentations by Sander van Maas, "Religion in a Broad Sense," Sher Doruff, "The Synaesthetic Biogram in Translocal Performance," and Aron Kibédi Varga (untitled). The third soirée was called *Concept and the Other Senses*, and the presenters were Margriet Schavemaker, "Performance and the Complicated Relation Between the Perceptual and the Conceptual," Maaike Bleeker, "Perceptual Concepts" and Vesna Madzoski, "'Blowin' in the Wind': LSD, The Sixties, and the Politics of the Nervous System." The fourth soirée was entitled *Skinaesthesia*, and involved presentations by Pieter Verstraete, "Skinaesthetic Imagination," Tarja Lane, "Cinema as Second Skin: Under the Membrane of Horror Film," Itay Sapir, "Seeing Texture, Touching Colour: Sensual Dialectics from 16th Century Venice to 20th Century Cool Britannia" and Tereza Havelkova, "Exploring Excess."

The presentations and discussion touched upon a wide variety of issues that cannot be easily summarized. Yet if one conclusion is to be drawn from the soirées, this might be that of a shift in the kind of questions that motivate and direct research into synesthesia from questions concerning the translation of one type of sensory experience into another (for example sound into color) or the relationship between two different types of sensory experience, towards questions concerning synesthesia as an intersensory experience, something in-between or even a borderline experience demanding a reconsideration of what is at stake in sense perception in general. This shift in focus also involves a rethinking of what exactly is synthesized in synesthesia (sound and vision, sound and shapes, percepts and concepts, time and space etc.) as well as the question how to understand the process of synthesizing and how to engage with it analytically.

**References**

Harrison, J. 2001. *Synaesthesia: The Strangest Thing*. Oxford: Oxford University Press.

Shaw-Miller, S. 2002. *Visible Deeds of Music*. New Haven: Yale University Press.

# SENSORY FORMATIONS SERIES

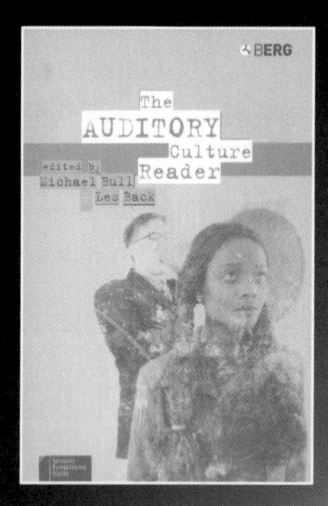

**Edited by Michael Bull & Les Back**
December 2003

HB 1 85973 613 0   £55.00   $99.95
PB 1 85973 618 1   £18.99   $32.95

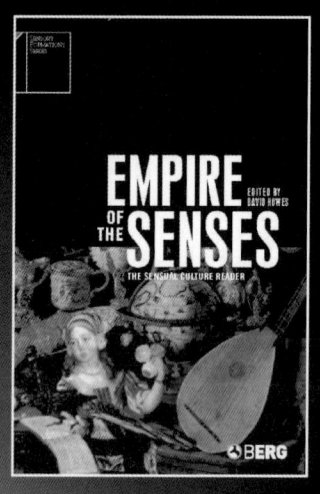

**Edited by David Howes**
December 2004

HB 1 85973 858 3   £60.00   $99.95
PB 1 85973 863 X   £19.99   $29.95

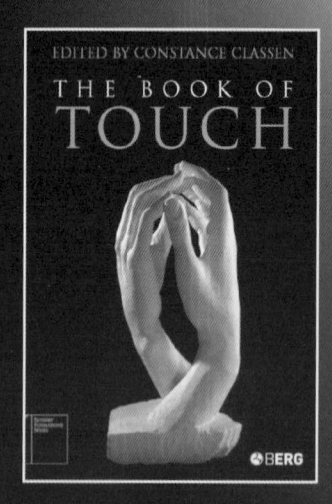

**Edited by Constance Classen**
July 2005

HB 1 84520 058 6   £55.00   $99.95
PB 1 84520 059 4   £19.99   $34.95

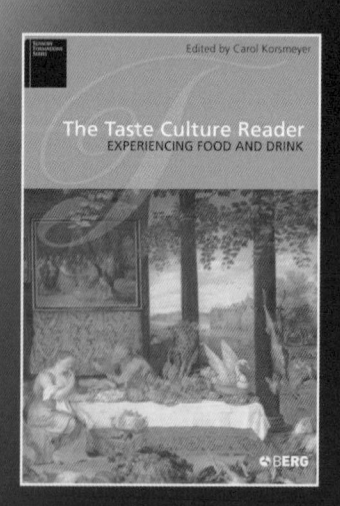

**Edited by Carolyn Korsmeyer**
August 2005

HB 1 84520 060 8   £55.00   $99.95
PB 1 84520 061 6   £19.99   $34.95

www.bergpublishers.com

# Senses of Identity

"A Sense of Identity" Lecture Series.
Convened by Shirley Ardener, Elisabeth Hsu,
Lidia Sciama and Ian Fowler, Institute of Social
and Cultural Anthropology, Oxford University,
Hilary Term 2006.

## Willow Sainsbury and Danny George

**Willow Sainsbury** holds a B.A. in Art and Archaeology from Princeton University and is currently pursuing research on "giftedness" in the context of psychiatric and neurological disorders – specifically, spatial awareness and dyslexia, in a M.Sc. program in Medical Anthropology at Oxford University. willow.sainsbury@magdalen.oxford.ac.uk

**Danny George** received his B.A. in English and Philosophy from The College of Wooster in Ohio. His research in the Oxford Medical Anthropology M.Sc. program concentrates on the human ecology of neurodegenerative diseases, and specifically Alzheimer's disease danny.george@hertford.ox.ac.uk

Each Friday morning from mid-January to mid-March 2006 the Institute of Social and Cultural Anthropology (ISCA) at Oxford University summoned up the senses with a seminar series titled "A Sense of Identity." The conveners, Shirley Ardener, Elisabeth Hsu, Lidia Sciama and Ian Fowler, had a vision for the series. They wanted speakers to explore how identity is experienced, shaped and expressed through one's senses and how, in culturally specific contexts, a given sense may acquire particular significance for the definition of identity.

Sara Davidmann from the University of the Arts in London began the series with a presentation of a select array of slides from her photographic portfolio. In a darkened lecture hall she shared dozens of images portraying the public and private manifestations of transsexual individuals struggling with their gender identity. The conventional role of vision in photography – the process by which an observer captures a subject – was inverted by Davidmann. She built up personal relationships with her participants and also assigned them agency in deciding their own visual representations. This artistic synergy allowed Davidmann to elucidate in great detail the limbo that transsexuals endure in modern society: "One door opens and another door closes, but the hallway is hell." She further explored the power of vision and visual representation to bring out the severe depression and angst suffered by transgendered individuals constrained by a society with rigid gender roles. However, there was also a celebration of transgender identity: this was achieved when the collaborative visual representations finally came to match the internal self images of the participants. Davidmann's seminar was a striking beginning to an exploration of the aesthetic dimensions of sensory experience.

In the following seminar, Adam Chau was concerned with articulating a sensory framework of and for social interaction. Chau's frustration at attempting to describe the social dynamics of the Black Dragon-King temple festival in contemporary China led him to invent a new vocabulary to describe the "red-hot fiery" collectivism he observed. Finding previous anthropological accounts of "collective action" lacking in sensation and dynamism, Chau played with neologisms such as "sensoric" and "socio-thermic affect" to convey the intensity of the ritual. As was evident from his made-up words, Chau conceptualized social cohesion as a variable form of "heat" generated between people who share the same physical space.

Whereas Chau's discussion of heat was largely ethereal, Gabi Alex examined the tangibility of touch in a seminar entitled, "'Touchability' and 'Untouchability' in India." In ethnographic accounts, "untouchability" has long been a dominant social trope. However, in her fieldwork, Alex focused on the extent to which touch is actually *integrated* into day-to-day social relations in India. Of particular interest to her was the role of touch in the process of growing up. Alex explored how tactile experience establishes strong symbolic boundaries and explained how categories of pure/impure are inculcated in children by adults. But she also captured the centrality of touch in children's formative years; according to her observations, no child was ever left alone, and children always sat in a way that left no space between them. Alex concluded that a subtle and important aesthetic of touch could be seen to undercut the paradigm of untouchability so dominant in Indian culture.

Elisabeth Ewart explored a similar dichotomy in her analysis of visibility and invisibility among the Panará of Central Brazil. Ewart examined the importance to the Panará of making social interactions visible to all. The circular layout of the village, whereby the houses fronted onto an open circle, created a central arena that made action and speech both visible and audible. The space at the back of the house that could not be witnessed by the whole community was only used for the family to exit and was unapproachable for any strangers. Ewart deduced that through hearing and seeing the community witnessed each other's activities and thus confirmed their humanness as opposed to the invisible and inaudible spirit world.

Clare Bryant explored how olfactory experience can also create a sense of community in her seminar, "Scenting a Subject." As Proust well knew, and other writers like him, smell, perhaps more intensively than any other sense, evokes memories. Bryant pointed out that we come to know our loved ones (and perhaps even our enemies) through their natural redolence, deodorants and perfumes. Even the slightest whiff of an airborne scent can give access to a repository of memories that contextualize one's own and others' identity in the present. Because of this intrinsic link between our sense of smell and the immediacy of memory, the olfactory aesthetic is indispensable to the achievement of human identity. On a lighter note, Bryant asked the audience to pay attention to smell and keep a "smell log." She evoked the range of smells found in parks and around Oxford that are frequently ignored in favor of artificial perfumes. 'She discussed the toxicity of some perfumes and how six scented products from talcum powder to soap are commonly used on newborn babies. The seminar drew from multiple sources and time periods to create an in depth look at smell.

Joy Adapon's seminar explored the question of how our sense of identity is mediated by our sense of taste. Adapon conducted her ethnography with a family in Mexico, keenly observing the centrality of cuisine to the maintenance of individual identity and social roles. Drawing on Bourdieu, she theorized that the way one tastes, perceives and learns to interact with food is shaped by one's habitus. And since we eat three meals a day, the centrality of food in our lives is a compelling subject for anthropological inquiry. Consequently, Adapon urged against devaluing taste as one of the "base senses," arguing that, from a cultural standpoint, food made in Mexican households is held in such high esteem as to be considered analogous to artwork. She observed that women who cooked delectable meals were ascribed social value and gained recognition for their culinary flair that would not otherwise been forthcoming in a machismo culture. Food is not simply utilitarian, she concluded: it is a social good that can be loaded with meanings that are salient to individuals across all cultures. As such, any anthropological exploration of identity must necessarily engage with the sense of taste.

In many ways, all the seminars in the series shared this richness. Overflowing audiences repeatedly filled the lecture hall each Friday morning, and lively discussions ensued after each presentation. Some of the other seminars, such as Roland Littlewood's on "The Blood of Christ," and Ian Flower on "Multi-sensorial Experience of Funerals in the Cameroon Grasslands," were thought-provoking presentations that should also be mentioned. All the seminars reminded us that the mind/body dichotomoy is a specious one since the senses essentially "feed" cognition and allow us to truly achieve human embodiment, and each posited an aesthetic attached to a particular corporeal sense. Diverse time periods were explored and commingled with intimate ethnographic accounts, cross disciplinary analysis and lively language and image to provide participants with a full-bodied understanding of the multiple "senses of identity."

# Textile

## The Journal of Cloth and Culture

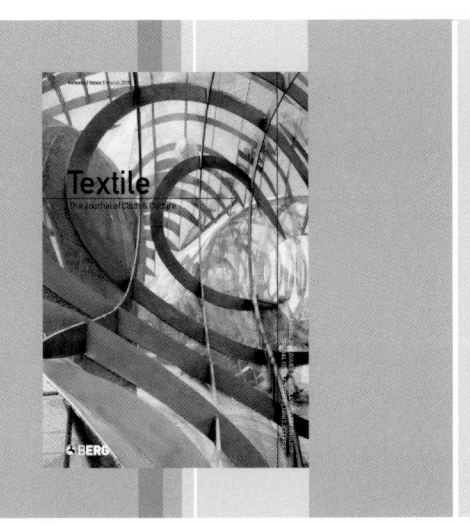

**Edited by Pennina Barnett,**
Goldsmiths College, University of London.
**Doran Ross,** UCLA Fowler Museum of Cultural History, Los Angeles.

*Winner of the 2005 ALPSP/ Charlesworth Award for Best New Journal*

'This journal has a lot going for it. It is easy to handle, well printed on good paper, imaginatively designed. Any university or college with an interest in textiles should subscribe to it and make it easily available. For individual scholars and makers, the journal provides a useful resource and will be a pleasure to collect and possess.'

**Times Higher Education**

Bringing together research in textiles in an innovative and distinctive academic forum, Textile provides a platform for points of departure between art and craft; gender and identity; cloth, body and architecture; labour and technology, techno-design and practice.

**Heavily illustrated, Full colour**

| TEXTILE | |
|---|---|
| ISSN 1475 9756 | |
| Individual Subscription | |
| Print only, does not include online access. | £46 / $79 |
| Institutional Print and Online | |
| Includes online access to all *Textile* back issues. | |
| Available through www.ingentaconnect.com | £125 / $225 |

**Indexed by:**
H.W. Wilson, Ebsco, IBSS (International Bibliography of Social Sciences), DAAI (Design and Applied Arts Index).

Published 3 times a year in March, July and November.

**BERG**

Order online at www.bergpublishers.com or call +44(0)1767 604951
Institutional subscriptions include online access through www.IngentaConnect.com
To order a sample copy please contact enquiry@bergpublishers.com
View issue 1.1 free online at www.ingentaconnect.com

# The Senses & Society

## Notes to Contributors

- Articles should be between 4,500 and 8,000 words (but not exceeding 8,000 words in length unless by prior agreement please).
- They must include a 30 word biography of the author(s) and a 200 abstract and 3 to 5 keywords.
- Interviews should also include an author biography.
- Exhibition and book reviews should be approximately 750 words, with occasional reviews running to 2,500 words.
- The Publishers will require a disk as well as a hard copy of any contributions.

From time to time, *Senses & Society* plans to produce special issues devoted to a single topic with a guest editor. Persons wishing to organize a topical issue are invited to submit a proposal which contains a 500-word description of the topic together with a list of potential contributors and paper subjects. Proposals are accepted only after a review by the Journal editors and in-house editorial staff at Berg Publishers.

## Manuscripts

- Manuscripts should be sent electronically in Microsoft Word with accompanying hard copy to:
  Dr Michael Bull, Managing Editor, The Senses and Society Journal, c/o Faculty of Arts and Humanities, University of Sussex, Falmer, Brighton, BN1 9RQ UK or to senses@sussex.ac.uk/M.Bull@sussex.ac.uk
- Manuscripts will be acknowledged and entered into the review process discussed below.
- Manuscripts without illustrations will not be returned unless the author provides a self-addressed stamped envelope.
- Submission of a manuscript to the journal will be taken to imply that it is not being considered elsewhere, in the same form, in any language, without the consent of the editor and publisher. It is a condition of acceptance by the editor of a manuscript for publication that the publishers automatically acquire the copyright of the published article throughout the world. Senses & Society does not pay authors for their manuscripts nor does it provide retyping, drawing, or mounting of illustrations.

## Style

- US spelling and mechanicals are to be used. Authors are advised to consult The Chicago Manual of Style (15th Edition) as a guideline for style. Webster's Dictionary is our arbiter of spelling. We encourage the use of major subheadings and, where appropriate, second-level subheadings.
- Manuscripts submitted for consideration as an article must contain:
  – a title page with the full title of the article, the author(s) name and address
  – a 30-word biography for each author.
- Do not place the author's name on any other page of the manuscript.

## Manuscript Preparation

- Manuscripts must be typed double-spaced (including quotations, notes and references cited), on one side only, with at least one-inch margins on standard paper using a typeface no smaller than 12pts.
- The original manuscript and a copy of the text on disk (please ensure it is clearly marked with the word-processing program that has been used) must be submitted, along with original photographs (to be returned).
- Authors should retain a copy for their records.
- Any necessary artwork must be submitted with the manuscript.

## Footnotes

- Footnotes appear as 'Notes' at the end of articles.
- Authors are advised to include footnote material in the text whenever possible.
- Notes are to be numbered consecutively throughout the paper and are to be typed double-spaced at the end of the text
- **(Please do not use any footnoting or end-noting programs which your software may offer as this text becomes irretrievably lost at the typesetting stage.)**

## References

- The list of references should be limited to, and inclusive of, those publications actually cited in the text.
- References are to be cited in the body of the text in parentheses with author's last name, the year of original publication, and page number—e.g. (Rouch 1958: 45).
- Titles and publication information appear as 'References' at the end of the article and should be listed alphabetically by author and chronologically for each author.
- References should be written in the following formats:
  Lewis, I.M. and C. Besteman. 1998. "Violence in Somalia: an Exchange." *Cultural Anthropology* 13(1): 100–14.
  Mayer, E. 1992. "Peru in Deep Trouble: Mario Vargas Llosa's 'Inquest in the Andes' Reexamined." In G.E. Marcus (ed.) *Rereading Cultural Anthropology*, pp.181–219. Durham: Duke University Press.
  Stoll, D. 1999. *Rigoberta Menchu and the Story of All Poor Guatemalans*. Boulder: Westview Press.
- Names of journals and publications should appear in full. Film and video information appear as 'Filmography'.
- References cited should be typed double-spaced on a separate page.
- References not presented in the style required will be returned to the author for revision.

## Tables

- All tabular material should be part of a separately numbered series of 'Tables'.
- Each table must be typed on a separate sheet and identified by a short descriptive title.
- Footnotes for tables appear at the bottom of the table.
- Marginal notations on manuscripts should indicate approximately where tables are to appear.

## Figures

All illustrative material: drawings, maps, diagrams, and photographs should be designated 'Figures'. They must be submitted in a form suitable for publication without redrawing.

- Drawings should be carefully done with India ink on either hard, white, smooth-surfaced board or good quality tracing paper. Ordinarily, computer-generated drawings are not of publishable quality.
- Photographs should be glossy prints and should be numbered on the back to key with captions. Whenever possible, photographs should be 8 × 10 inches.
- The publishers also encourage artwork to be submitted as scanned files (300dpi or above ONLY) on disc or via email.
- All figures should be numbered consecutively.
- All captions should be typed double-spaced on a separate page.
- Marginal notations on manuscripts should indicate approximately where figures are to appear.
- While the editors and publishers will use all reasonable care in protecting all figures submitted, they cannot assume responsibility for their loss or damage. Authors are discouraged from submitting rare or non-replaceable materials. It is the author's responsibility to secure written copyright clearance (for both print and online usage) on all photographs and drawings that are not in the public domain.

## Criteria for Evaluation

Senses & Society is a refereed journal. Manuscripts will be accepted only after review by both the editors and anonymous reviewers deemed competent to make professional judgments concerning the quality of the manuscript.

## Reprints for Authors

Twenty-five reprints of author's articles will be provided to the author free of charge. Additional reprints may be purchased upon request.